THE CLUELESS DAD'S GUIDE TO FIRST-TIME PREGNANCY

Things I Learned That Every Expectant Father Should Know

Dwayne Mills

© Copyright 2020

All rights reserved.

Disclaimer Notice

Please note the information contained within this document is for educational and entertainment purposes only. All effort has been executed to present accurate, up to date, and reliable, complete information. No warranties of any kind are declared or implied. Readers acknowledge that the author is not engaging in the rendering of legal, financial, medical or professional advice. The content within this book has been derived from the author's personal experiences and various sources. Please consult a licensed professional before attempting any techniques outlined in this book.

By reading this document, the reader agrees that under no circumstances is the author responsible for any losses, direct or indirect, which are incurred as a result of the use of the information contained within this document, including, but not limited to, — errors, omissions, or inaccuracies.

Table of Contents

Introduction

So here we go. I hope you are strapped in. It is about to get messy in all the best and beautiful ways life knows how to be. On the basis you are reading this humble work of nonfiction, the chances are that you are; potentially collaborating with someone to create a little bundle of joy in the future; the proud (yet possibly terrified) partner of someone who is expecting your first little bundle of joy; possibly an uber-planner wanting to make sure you are ridiculously prepared for the job title of "Dad" someday in the future; and or, perhaps are just slightly eccentric, with a niche sense of humor, manifesting itself in a deep appreciation for the comedy of errors that is the male cohort of Homo sapiens preparing themselves for the role of being a father.

Whichever group(s) of audience you fall into, my hope is that through recounting some of my own journey on the way to becoming a father for the first time, I can help the reader feel encouraged, more relaxed, more knowledgeable and hopefully less anxious, about what is both an indescribably wonderful process, and yet a very daunting undertaking. Further, it is worth highlighting that being a Clueless Dad may well be a comedy of errors, but if played correctly, it can also be a journey of growth that challenges any epic Shakespearian pursuit. If played badly, however, it can have many elements of a Greek tragedy. There is no doubt that the Clueless Dad is embarking on his own quest and as a result, we hope that some of the content, stories, and tips, will help them along the way to avoid many dangers, conquer any foes and vanquish their demons.

On the road to becoming a father for the first time, you will likely be exposed to a plethora of strong emotions. Depending on the route you take, the personalities involved, the unique blend of concocted hormones, the time you invest in preparation, and the mental health of those involved, it can be relatively smooth, or very tempestuous. At times during this voyage, you may want to laugh and cry, shout and scream (while quickly duck flying objects aimed at your head), hug and hold, and even possibly run and hide - hopefully not, but it is not uncommon.

The good news is that no two journeys are the same, nor is one better or worse than the other. Like anything in nature, there is a spectrum and while some people experience breezy pregnancies, some people emerge feeling like they have done a tour of duty. The important thing is for you to know that before you jump out of the pregnancy plane some 10,000 feet above the earth, there is always support and help available for pretty much any scenario, no matter where you fall on nature's spectrum. Furthermore, suppose you end up towards the tempestuous end of this experience. In that case, you can weather most conditions if approached with a level of selflessness, mutual respect, self-care, and an openness to learn and develop.

While there is no one-size-fits-all recipe for success, it will make you grow stronger as a couple, a man in your own right, and, ideally, a competent father. We all have a duty to try and reduce society's "daddy issues" for both our men and women. I have a suspicion it would have a huge positive impact on the running of the world, general happiness, the environment, economic prosperity, the way we treat each other, and the human race's true ability to create things of meaning and value. And so with that as a lofty but worthy, overarching goal, what ensues in the following chapters is my best efforts to get the average man on the street ready for the seismic shock and indelible experience of being a father.

Every part of society needs its heroes and role models. The category of being a father is no different. I admire anyone who excels in any chosen endeavor, especially one where success should lead to a better, more balanced, and secure youth of tomorrow. However, this book is dedicated to the common man, who may need a little extra help and encouragement. This book was written for the men who, on the face of it, may seem to be excited, but only a few millimeters below the surface, are feeling weak at the knees from the gravity of the situation. This book was written for the man who really wants to be supportive to his wonderful partner, but maybe sheltering deep fears of never being able to go to steak night or watch the game with his buddies EVER AGAIN!

I feel qualified to write about this because I was that guy. I am definitely more qualified to write this tale than I was ever qualified to be a father. But, that is the beauty of the fatherhood journey. If you are willing to do some (any) work, you can most likely figure it out. During my fatherhood apprenticeship, I made a ton of mistakes. I was very naive, grossly underestimated the task's size, and all-around underprepared, but it didn't stop me. This was sometimes through trial and error, and sometimes through luck. Other times, it was because I had decent support and access to useful information. But throughout those moments of tumult and stress, I took comfort in the fact that through history, way less qualified people had made it work. I could relate to this even within my own family and close friendship groups. Some of these men I referred to didn't just make it work, they had been great fathers against all odds. As an extension of this line of thinking, the fact you are alive today means someone managed to raise you and your parents, and their parents, and so on, back until our caveman ancestors and beyond. I don't know if the parenting was always good, and my sneaking suspicion is that mothers typically should take more of the credit, but we all made it to today. If we start with that fact as the lowest hurdle, there is wide open space to be an awesome dad, irrespective of our pervasive primitive tendencies.

So with that snapshot of how this book came to be and the various people it was designed to help, it is worth highlighting what else you can expect from it. Yes, it covers a collection of weird and wonderful tales of the things I learned, a few items I should have pre-learned, and some key insights and tools that can be employed to smooth out any potholes along the way.

I am not a healthcare professional. Furthermore, while I will be touching on several medical areas for your awareness, none of my layman observations or opinions should be considered any form of advice. I am sure it goes without saying, but if you or your partner have any physical or mental concerns, you should consult a healthcare professional at your earliest convenience.

In closing, despite some puerile humor (a trait I actually credit getting through the birth of my two children relatively unscathed with), I hope you find the messages contained herein to be useful, enjoyable, and worthwhile. For the reader's benefit, I have tried to operate with honesty, integrity, and transparency. Furthermore, despite the unavoidable truth that I am recounting my lived experiences, which will inherently contain my biases, I have tried to remain as balanced and objective as humanly possible. Each journey was different in their own way, but alike at their purest core. There is a natural inclination to entertain with any written content, but I have worked hard not to be sensationalist and or inauthentic. This is because, if the messages in this book genuinely apply to you, then behind all the words and hyperbole, the responsibility you are assuming is one of the largest and most real responsibilities you can take on. It should not be taken lightly, and I respect you for taking it on. Yet, at the same time, it doesn't mean it can't be enjoyable, fulfilling, and character building.

Chapter 1

Honey We're Pregnant

"I'm pregnant" is in the top five most impactful life sentences, in my opinion. It could actually be in the top three. Depending on your own personal journey, it can be one of the most magical, scary, vexing, and exhilarating sentences that you can hear. Chances are that when you are on the receiving end of such notification (and you have verified that you are the partner in crime, so to speak), you will experience elements of several of those emotions and an abundance of other ones. While you will undoubtedly be excited, you will likely also be a little overwhelmed, no matter how much you have prepared or thought about it. Some emotions might be a little uncomfortable or stressful, and let me be clear, that is totally natural and ok. Hopefully, you feel nothing but pure positivity and the joy of anticipation, but if you are in the more challenging area of your emotional responses, do not worry. It is very typical. Over time, if you feel like you are lingering too long in this less than optimistic region of your thoughts and feelings, it is undoubtedly worth seeking the help of a health professional.

You are Never Fully Prepared for "I'm pregnant"

My experience will be different from yours, but let me recount my "I'm pregnant" moment. At the time, I was on holiday in Italy for a close friend's wedding. My girlfriend (now wife) had returned home to get back to work, and I was spending a few extra days in Tuscany with some friends. As you do in the middle of an Italian summer, we went into town to check out the architecture and the local Tuscan wines. I was in the middle of a fun afternoon with the groom, minding my own business, and enjoying a couple of glasses of pinot grigio in the sun when she called.

"Are you alone?" Sounds ominous I thought.

"No. I'm with ... (let's call him Billy)".

"Can you get away from him?" Doubly ominous.

"Not really. You want to tell me what's going on?" I did have a little flash of panic that something had gone wrong.

"I need to tell you something." Oh my gosh, she's changed her mind. She's upgraded to a proper alpha male and I am about to be put in the recycling bin.

"Go on then."

"I'm pregnant".

And there we are! Brief, innocent, but forever life-changing. That short but very impactful exchange of words had me in a total spin. I was delighted, stunned, relieved (that my split-second alpha-male upgrade was a figment of my imagination) and generally flooded with a multitude of emotions. I was probably quite lucky I had been sampling some local alcoholic fayre, as I was relaxed and in a good mood. At a rare but selfless level, I was also so, so happy for my lady. With the advent of this news, we had taken the first step towards making this life plan a reality. However, it is important to be aware of a couple of things at this exciting but nascent part of the pregnancy journey.

How to Deal with the Potential Risk of Miscarriage

Now I was lucky. Despite the challenges we experienced while getting pregnant, we had a relatively easy pregnancy. Not everyone does for a host of reasons, so it is worth deconstructing my "I'm pregnant" skit for the reader's benefit. In my scenario, Billy was a great comrade to experience that situation with. At the time, he had a 2-year-old boy and could relate to my situation. However, with the benefit of hindsight, I would have preferred to find out in isolation had I not been so caught by surprise. This is due to the sad but undeniable fact that just getting pregnant is not a guarantee that you will produce a perfectly healthy baby. In the same way that Mother Nature does not always comply with the wishes of longing parents, she can also be a little cruel in the early stages of pregnancy. While the numbers vary across regions, approximately 15-25% of all identified pregnancies will end in a miscarriage on average. This rate is actually estimated to be higher when including pregnancies, where they were not recognized or identified. For example, this type of miscarriage occurs when a woman miscarries before she even misses a menstrual period and or realizes she is pregnant.

A miscarriage is typically defined as the loss of a fetus before the 20th week of pregnancy. As a result, it is important to understand that it is better not to tell anyone that your partner is pregnant until you are out of the higher risk period. There is no scientifically identified "right time" to announce a pregnancy. The dangers of a miscarriage start to diminish significantly at the end of the first trimester, around 10-12 weeks in. We waited until 12 weeks. Bear in mind that your partner may not even start "showing" until the third, fourth, or fifth month. This means that no-one will be able to tell she is even pregnant until around that time. As such, it should cause you no disruption to keep that cheeky little piece of intel to yourself until the appropriate time.

As a side note, we had several friends experience the painful speed bump of a miscarriage. I hope no one reading this book will end up in that category. However, as I came to understand the maths and probabilities around the frequency of miscarriages, I realized that they are pretty common. We think they aren't because, like many painful events in life, people prefer not to discuss them, but they are. Remember, 15-25% is relatively high. Given this rate, I think that they should be discussed more as a way to de-stigmatize this unfortunate twist of nature and, where needed, lend emotional support. I appreciate that as a man, I have limited claim over this subject as it is the woman's body that is directly affected. Still, miscarriages can be painful for expectant fathers too. In addition, as with many upsetting events, I think the more people can speak through their challenges and see that they are not alone, the quicker the route to grieving and healing.

Keep Your Powder Dry

Going early on the announcement of the pregnancy is similar to going early on the disclosure of the name. I have had a few friends (typically men) who went early on disclosing the name and it was a mistake. It was not meant with any malintent and was often done so out of some sort of childish excitement, but it is often dimly looked upon, particularly when not authorized by your partner. You will be amazed at how many times the name will change, particularly in the final trimester. If you take any advice from one new father to a soon to be one, do not underestimate this little point of decorum. Try and hold on, because if you don't, it can easily backfire and upset your number one collaborator. The same can be said for the man. I saw a male colleague of mine treat the name "launch codes" like the highest level security clearance possible to the atom bomb, only to find out that his wife's entire circle of friends already knew the preferred name. This was not well received. Particularly when he found out his wife had changed her mind (again) and without informing him. The bottom line around sensitive pregnancy-related disclosures to friends and family is, wait until you know it is appropriate. How will you know if it is appropriate? Asking your partner is a good place to start.

What Type of Father Do You Want to Be?

In order to help you make the transition and acclimate to this new "you," with all the increased sense of awareness, responsibility, and expectation for the future, it is worth engaging in some self-analysis around what you expect from this journey and why you expect it. It can help to speak to your parents to understand what they were like and how they handled it. Naturally, it makes sense to try and review your father's experience, if possible, and see if the way he felt and behaved during his Clueless Dad journey resonates with your outlook and blueprint for yourself. This advice may seem a little obscure, but I guarantee you that you will not be fully prepared for this experience no matter how much planning you have done. As such, the quickest way to get ready mentally and emotionally is to spend time really contemplating what is truly important to you, what is critical for the journey, and what might be superfluous or not as important as you first thought.

For example, you may think it is important to conceal your emotions to appear strong for your partner. Or, you may deem it necessary to tell your parents that your partner is pregnant early on because they are your parents. Both examples may seem perfectly reasonable. However, what if by appearing strong, you actually appear unemotional at a time when she needs emotional support. Or in the latter scenario, by telling your parents early, you build a sense of expectation and with it an implied pressure with such an expectation, only to experience the small but stinging setback of a miscarriage. These examples could be any number of potential hiccups in this early stage of pregnancy. The main message here is that you can short cut risks of misfortune by spending quality time reflecting on your priorities, considering your motivations and behavioral drivers, and testing your assumptions.

Don't Freak Out

Aside from the mental upgrade you will experience and the expansion of perception that comes with the knowledge that you will likely be a new Father in eight to nine months, it is also worth addressing some of the more common concerns. Common questions are as follows: -

"Will I be any good?"

"Is this the end of my freedom?"

"How on earth am I going to be able to pay for an additional dependent?"

"How do I make sure I am prepared mentally and emotionally for this?"

"How can I make sure that I am both a decent husband or partner, and father?"

"I hope I don't drop the baby!"

"What if my son or daughter doesn't like me?"

"Do I want to know the sex of the baby?"

"When can you even find out the sex of the baby?"
(It's 16 - 20 weeks).

"Will my inlaws be a pain during this process?"

"Will my inlaws be able to help during this
process?"

"What shall we call it, if it's a boy?"

"What shall we call the baby, if it's a girl?"

"I know what men are like, please don't be a girl!"

"I don't mean that, I will be happy either gender,
just as long as it's healthy!"

"What would we do if the baby has health problems?"

"When do I start antenatal classes?"

"Do I have to go to antenatal classes?"

"Of course I want to go to antenatal classes!"

The list could go on into eternity. We, humans, have a tendency to be overthinkers, and sometimes, although it is hard to admit, sometimes we aren't super-rational. However, as highlighted above, these types of questions are all perfectly natural and normal. We cover some of these questions as we work through the book, and other questions where there is not a prescriptive solution, we suggest ways to think about getting to a personal answer for the reader. The overarching principle of this book is to keep reminding you that you are not alone in your hopes and fears regarding being an extraordinary father. There are often solutions to challenges and if you are uncertain about anything, there are billions of men who either are or have been in your position and survived.

What Comes Next?

Having covered the initial excitement and potential surprise of this joyous news, we start to look at ways to take care of your partner in the following chapter(s). We also look at the equally important ways for you to look after yourself. We then look at some of the financial considerations and start to take you through the journey on a month by month basis. Throughout this process, we make suggestions on tools you can use, tips that may help, and other potential resources you can lean on to keep up the momentum.

Chapter 2

How to Take Care of Her Physically

Looking after your partner during their pregnancy is probably the most important role. You need to be very cognizant that your partner is undergoing a massive change in their body, which could impact everything from craving the most out-of-character foods known to man (like really strange), to their self-image, to their sense of wellbeing and safety, to their feelings about you. When reflecting upon my own experience to a friend of mine, I likened it to taking a voyage at sea. You hope for good weather, but be aware and prepared that it could also be stormy and turbulent. That said, I tried to retain two simple truths; storms always pass, even the worst ones; and the better prepared and more knowledgeable you are during a period of turbulence, the more likely you are to emerge from it safely and unscathed. My overarching observation is that like anything important and valuable, it may take some hard work and commitment, but the payoff will always be worth it. So having said that, let's jump into some of the areas of physical health where you can really help to make sure she is being healthy and looking after herself.

Sleep

Needless to say, growing a human in your belly is no small feat. Before you can even visibly tell that she is pregnant, the conception and subsequent gestation of your special little one will start to increasingly make demands on your partner. I often observed that many of the actions an expecting mother should take during her pregnancy resembled closely the necessary activities for the newborn child. First of all, naps are like nature's magical elixir for repairing and regenerating a pregnant woman's body. Some practitioners advise taking a nap at lunch and before dinner, but also to get into the habit of taking 10-20 minute power-naps whenever it is possible. Unsurprisingly, a good night's sleep is also deeply beneficial. Your lady should be trying to aim for 8 hours per night and you should be encouraging her to target this as well (at least in the first two trimesters, before the discomfort and overall size of the newborn starts to disrupt sleep in the third trimester). Selfishly, sleep will also make life easier for you as well. It is amazing how a decent sleep can take the sting out of any tough relationship situations, particularly during a pregnancy. In this set of circumstances however, it will not only help your partner's mood, but also see it as an investment in the development of the health and wellbeing of your unborn daughter or son.

In the same vein as napping and sleep, it is also worth spending the time to encourage your lady to simply rest periodically throughout the day. If you are married to Wonderwoman and she has trouble slowing down, she may well start to find that her swollen ankles and back pain become more than slight irritations and turn into proper speed bumps. It is better to take a load off and decompress during little intervals throughout the day, rather than let any discomfort build up and boil over. You should support this as much as is reasonably possible. That said it can be difficult if your partner is still working during her pregnancy. It may be that you can only oblige her on weekends at the start.

Food and Drink

Hydration is a simple, but very effective tool to support a woman in the early stages of pregnancy. This is because it keeps the blood properly hydrated and therefore helps with circulation. Not only does it reduce the toll on the woman, but it also helps with the development of the baby, who is also accordingly well hydrated through the mother's bloodstream. The exact guidance varies, but if you can support your partner to drink between eight and ten cups of water per day, that is ideal.

Drinking lots of water may seem quite elementary, but it is worth remembering that it can also lower the propensity for cramps and other strains. In addition, drinking a lot of water can help the body synthesize the increased supply of strong hormones, which can make the skin more sensitive and lead to stretch marks and itchiness. Plain still water is best, but bear in mind that if your partner is experiencing morning sickness they may have trouble holding it down. If this is the case, it is typically suggested that some sort of natural sweetener (like honey, sugar) can be added to make it more palatable. Alternatively, sucking ice cubes and or drinking fresh fruit juice can also help. I took to squeezing fresh orange juice for my wife, which I also managed to get in on as well.

Newly pregnant women will be advised to maintain a healthy and balanced diet in order for them to keep their blood sugar in appropriate levels. It will likely be suggested to your partner that she eats frequent smaller portion sizes, with a focus on protein, foods rich in natural fiber (fruits and vegetables, ideally 5 servings a day), and unprocessed starchy foods for energy (potatoes, rice, bread, and pasta). Healthcare practitioners will likely suggest avoiding high-calorie foods and drinks that are fried and or, high in sugars and fats. If you are able to help her through this by shopping and preparing for these types of meals, you will be a hero.

Generally speaking, pregnant women can continue to eat meat and poultry as normal, but with some considerations listed below in "What not to eat". As an extension of this, fish can also be a great source of nutrients, particularly as a source of protein, iron, and zinc, all of which help your unborn child's development and growth. In addition, the omega 3 fatty acids in fish can help both the baby's brain development, as well as the brain health of the pregnant mother. Furthermore, Omega 3 fatty acids are thought to help offset low mood and or depression which can be very valuable if your partner happens to be susceptible to these challenges during pregnancy.

As a general rule, if you are trying to help your partner add seafood to her diet, you should be helping her to include varieties that not only contain high levels of omega-3 fatty acids but importantly, low levels of mercury. It is worth noting however, that healthcare professionals go a step further and recommend avoiding specific types of fish due to high levels of mercury. This is because mercury can have a detrimental effect on your baby's development and in particular, their nervous system. We discuss several of these underwater rogues as well in the following section of "What not to eat".

Some examples of recommended seafood include, salmon, tilapia, pollock, catfish, trout, pacific mackerel (as opposed to king mackerel), sardines, anchovies, herrings, and canned light tuna. Albacore tuna and tuna steaks are typically recommended to be restricted to 6 ounces per week. As a general rule, most shellfish are acceptable as long as they have been thoroughly cooked. For example, no sloppy, slippery and salty oysters for a while (unless they have been thoroughly cooked). If you are being Gordon Ramsay in the kitchen for your partner after a long day, it is worth keeping in mind that the Mayo Clinic says fish should be cooked to an internal temperature of at least 145°F (63°C).

If, like me, you find adhering to a balanced diet hard at the best of times, let alone helping someone else do it, the process can be quite taxing. However, if you view it as another investment in your unborn child's health and potentially a controlled health experiment that you can run on yourself, it can help with the motivation and getting into a decent routine around mealtimes.

What Not to Eat

What not to eat while pregnant is nearly more important than what to eat. Some of these items may seem very obscure and therefore, supporting her abstinence may seem effortless. However, there are a couple of guilty pleasures that are better left alone during pregnancy, but that can be hard to forgo if they are part of your lady's (or your own) eating routine. We use guidance from the UK's NHS (National Health Service) and NCT (National Childbirth Trust) to shape this discussion.

Raw eggs are a definite no-no (I told you some of the items weren't too hard to consider giving up). More specifically, if she eats eggs regularly, they need to be cooked until all the whites and yolks are solid. If they are not, she risks exposure to salmonella which is dangerous anyway but presents a much more acute risk for pregnant women.

Products containing liver and pâté should be disregarded. This is because not only can they contain a lot of vitamin A, which can be detrimental to an unborn child, but they can also contain listeria bacteria. Listeria bacteria is also commonly found in deli meats and unpasteurized dairy products and does not usually cause much harm to mature, healthy people. However, listeria bacteria can cause listeria infection, which can have serious consequences for pregnant women and be fatal to unborn babies and or newborns. This is due to the woman's weakened immune system and the unborn child's unformed immune system.

To expand on the specific types of dairy products that should be left alone, you need to help your partner avoid any raw (unpasteurized) milk. If she can't do without it, then it should be boiled to remove any bacteria first. Your pregnant partner should also avoid unpasteurized cheeses. These include products made from soft goats' cheese, like for example, chèvre. She will also have to omit mold-ripened cheeses like brie and camembert and or soft blue-veined cheese like roquefort and or

Danish blue. Again, these precautions are to avoid any clashes with listeria bacteria.

 If this is a little confusing and leaves your cheese strategy in chaos, bear in mind that in the US and other Western countries with similar food types, most cheeses are made using pasteurized milk which kills the bacteria. While you should always check the label and instructions for safety, most supermarket cheeses are safe to eat, outside the types listed above.

Uncooked or rare meat must also be avoided. All meat and poultry need to be cooked to a "well done" level, ensuring it has no traces of blood or pink juice. It is recommended that particular care is taken when preparing pork, sausages, minced meat and poultry. This is to limit the potential risk of salmonella, coliform bacteria and or coming down with toxoplasmosis. This last term is a fancy word for contracting an infection from the *Toxoplasma* parasite that is in the meat and has not been completely eliminated by thoroughly cooking.

I have to admit, I was surprised by the risks of toxoplasmosis. I was surprised because it suggested that there should have been an ongoing risk to people who eat rare or raw meat when they are not pregnant. It turns out that this risk is actually continually present for those people who eat meat. However, a healthy human's immune system will typically keep the parasite at bay and stop it from causing sickness. When a woman is pregnant however, she has a weakened immune system and therefore needs to exercise caution.

I mentioned deli meats above in the same category as the pates and livers. These products are also often referred to as cold meats and typically comprise products like salami, prosciutto and chorizo. These types of meats are most often cured and fermented, as opposed to cooked. This means that they can carry risks of both listeria and toxoplasmosis. Some pre-packed products like ham or corned beef are considered safe, but you or your partner should always check the packaging and instructions as a first-line safety precaution.

As set out earlier, some types of fish are also omitted from the recommended pregnancy diet and in particular, any raw fish (think sushi or ceviche), for obvious reasons. It is also suggested that expecting mothers steer clear of large predatory fish such as swordfish, shark, king mackerel and tilefish. This is predominantly to avoid mercury. Mercury in fish doesn't typically impact adults. Yet, like many of the risks we have covered, it comes into focus during pregnancy and is best given a little dietary vacation until your little one has landed and you can start to return to your normal eating patterns (if the term normal is even possible with a newborn).

I left the most contentious item until last, coffee. If you are like me or your partner is like my wife, coffee is like oxygen for you and you can barely think straight until you have had that caffeine injection each morning. Sadly, this magical little drink, and to a lesser extent teas containing caffeine are required to be reined in during pregnancy. This is predominantly because consuming large amounts of caffeine while pregnant can lead to miscarriage and low birthweight for the baby.

The good news is that your partner doesn't have to cut out caffeine completely (although my wife did - again, to be completely safe). However, she typically shouldn't drink more than 200mg a day, which is approximately 0.007 ounces. If these amounts mean nothing to you, like they did to me, then here are some reference points. A mug of filter coffee has around 140mg, a mug of instant coffee has approximately 100mg, a mug of tea typically has 75mg and a can of cola has around 40mg. It is worth remembering that chocolate can contain caffeine, as can some herbal teas such as green or matcha tea.

It can be a pain in the proverbial backside to keep a record of your lady's caffeine intake. Therefore, some simple rules on daily consumption can take away some of the ambiguity and irritation that micromanaging this area can bring. I would still suggest that avoiding caffeine completely is the best choice, just to be on the safer side.

Dangers of Toxoplasmosis

Having mentioned the threat of toxoplasmosis above, I wanted to spend a short amount of time on this subject while it is fresh in your head, and before the next section. If you think toxoplasmosis sounds a little far-fetched, the Centers for Disease Control and Prevention (CDC) states that there are 40 million people in the United States with Toxoplasmosis. This is over 10% of the population so it is worth at least knowing about it.

In addition to the food types listed above, it is worth also being aware that Toxoplasmosis can be contracted by swallowing the parasite through contact with cat feces. Now before you stop reading thinking this is ridiculous, the CDC lists accidental ingestion may happen after; cleaning a cat's litter box; touching or ingesting anything that has come into contact with the *Toxoplasma* parasite and or somehow accidentally consuming contaminated soil (potentially after gardening or eating unwashed fruits and vegetables from the garden). Yes, no sane person is going to be in the habit of eating their pet cat feces. But bear in mind, these little critters may also be carrying these bacteria innocently and unknowingly as a result of their own personal hygiene regimes. They can also carry the parasites under their nails from standing in a litter and spread them. Cats can get a rough reputation when it comes to toxoplasmosis. Our feline friends are viewed a little bit as a pariah in this area, whereas their canine counterparts are given a free ride as they are less susceptible to the *Toxoplasma* parasite. In fact, dogs are not natural hosts, and are generally infected via consuming cat feces. Cats on the other hand are definitive hosts of this parasite.

The good news is that if you are cohabiting with a purring, fuzzy little bundle of joy, you don't have to get rid of them just because your partner is pregnant. However, it does require an increased level of vigilance and hygiene. I would recommend a quick review of the CDC's guidelines. As an example, you may need to man up and commit to changing the kitty litter for the foreseeable future 100% of the time. Similarly, you may need to increase the frequency of this as the *Toxoplasma* parasite doesn't become infectious until one to five days after the cat has done its poop. You may also need to only feed your cat dry or canned food, avoiding raw (another way of saying "caught outside") or undercooked meats and ideally you keep your cat away from strays and specifically kittens.

In addition to the various actions listed above, there are several ways to ensure a symbiotic relationship between you, your lady and your cat(s) during the pregnancy. It just requires some clear ground rules, mutual respect and a willingness from all parties to compromise and work together.

Vegan or Vegetarian?

Maintaining a vegetarian or vegan diet during pregnancy is very possible, but it does require a little extra effort. This presents a great opportunity for the man in the relationship to sparkle as a chivalrous knight in shining armor, dashingly supporting their partner's food plan. In order to do so, it is worth knowing what we are aiming for. As a simple starting point, we want to zero in on iron, calcium, vitamin B12 and vitamin D, amongst other nutrients and vitamins (which we discuss later). Most of these are found in meat and fish, which can be a little problematic if you typically do not eat these items. While we would suggest you speak to your doctor to discuss how best to respect your dietary preferences, while still getting the right amount of nutrition, the following suggestions are here to help guide you, in helping to guide her. For ease of understanding, where we refer to options for vegans, we assume that for the most part, that these food types are inherently acceptable for vegetarians.

If your partner chooses a vegetarian diet, eggs are good for iron. For vegans, iron can be sourced via tofu, pulses, dark green vegetables (spinach, collard greens, kale), sauerkraut, oatmeal and in some cases, dried fruits (apricots, prunes, raisins and figs).

It is well known that calcium is found in dairy products such as milk and cheese. However, for vegans getting enough calcium can be challenging. That said, dark green vegetables are a good source, as well as calcium enriched plant-based milk including soy, rice and oat. Calcium can also be found in certain types of bread, sesame seeds, tahini, dried fruits and calcium-set tofu.

Vitamin B12 is found in dairy products and eggs for vegetarians. For vegans, they can source B12 from enriched breakfast cereals and plant-based milk drinks, like soy. However, it is often recommended that vegans also take a supplement as well to ensure they are consuming enough B12.

Vitamin D is only found in a small number of foods, but is a very important nutrient. For vegetarians, it is found in egg yolks. For vegans, it can be found in vitamin D enriched breakfast cereals and most non-dairy fat spreads or butter substitutes. Given the importance of vitamin D for your partner, she should get advice on taking an ongoing vitamin D supplement. This is particularly relevant over winter, as sunlight is a strong source of vitamin D.

For those who do not eat fish, you can help your lady consume omega-3 fatty acids from several plant-based sources. For example, flaxseed (whether ground or in oil form), canola oil, walnuts, sunflower seeds and soybeans (edamame) are all great sources of omega-3s. For vegetarians, yogurt, milk and eggs can be fortified with omega-3 fatty acids. You can supplement omega-3s but this can be tricky as they typically contain fish oil, so depending on your preference, it pays to take medical advice and be vigilant.

I understand that this can be a little overwhelming for a Clueless Dad who may not have been completely on top of his nutrient and vitamin game to begin with. To be constantly worrying about getting enough of the necessary food types can possibly seem like a chore, particularly if it doesn't come naturally to you. However, it is one of the simplest ways in which you (with mother nature's help) can support your lady and your unborn little one through this period. A little extra awareness and support from you to make sure your partner is benefitting from a nutritious diet can make a significant difference.

Morning Sickness

When talking about what to eat and not to eat, it is worth spending a little time on morning sickness and ways to deal with it. Morning sickness is a strange creature. It can really impact (and in some cases, not impact) people in very different ways and with varying levels of severity. There is no singular cause, but it is generally accepted that the change in hormones during pregnancy is a main culprit. The good news is that morning sickness is common and will usually pass without leaving any impact on the pregnant mother or unborn child. That said, it can be very unpleasant and wreak havoc on your endeavor to help your partner eat well and stay hydrated.

The most common symptoms are nausea and vomiting. These symptoms are often set off by certain smells, types of foods, heat and excess saliva, to name a few. Sometimes, there is no trigger which can be even more elusive. While morning sickness will usually abate after the first trimester, you should get your partner to the doctor or other health care provider if the nausea and or vomiting is severe and or she cannot keep down liquids. Dehydration for obvious reasons is concerning as we discussed the importance of the expecting mother drinking enough water earlier. Other symptoms which likely necessitate a trip to the clinic or surgery include, if your partner is having trouble passing small amounts of urine or it is particularly dark in color; if she is dizzy or faint when she stands up; and she has a racing heart or palpitations.

Being that there is no specific cause and no specific treatment, it is hard to help your partner avoid morning sickness. Instead, you need to try and avoid the triggers that you both become aware of and try to lend a helping hand during the times when the symptoms are giving her trouble. If she can identify the smells that are setting her off, or the types of foods that are causing her to be repulsed, then it is obvious that you should eliminate them. However, in some cases, where she has particular cravings or more pleasant associations with certain food types, you can double down on those. These often may be spicy or sweet, or potentially more left field, think anchovies or pickled gherkins. Whatever her preference, the positive association she has with the food type can mentally offset the physical feelings of discomfort and queasiness. As a final thought, the Mayo Clinic also highlights that excessive fatigue can trigger morning sickness, so I refer back to the section around resting and napping.

Vitamins and Supplements

In the section above, we covered several vitamins and nutrients (iron, calcium, vitamin B12 and vitamin D). That was discussed looking through the frame of a vegetarian or vegan diet. In this section, we spend a little time looking at some recommended dosages as well as, looking at other necessary supplements that you should be aware of and gently encouraging your partner to consume, regardless of diet.

Number one in our list is folic acid. This nutrient is a rockstar supplement that is recommended to be taken while trying to get pregnant and then for the first 12 weeks of the pregnancy. Folic acid is a B vitamin that helps the body grow new cells. It is interesting to note that folic acid is actually a synthetic form of folate. A woman can consume folic acid via foods in which they have been enriched with the supplement. These include breads, pastas, rice and some breakfast cereals. It is also found in spinach, beans, asparagus and to a lesser extent, in oranges and peanuts.

Our good friends at the CDC (when they aren't accusing people of eating cat feces) recommend that women of conception age take 400mcg (micrograms) of folic acid daily. However, it can be as high as 1,000mcg. Folic acid helps protect the baby from developmental issues and in particular, neural tube defects which lead to heart breaking defects of the brain and spine. Fun fact: the recommended dosage increases to 600 mcg in the second and third trimesters, and then drops to 500 mcg while breastfeeding.

While you consider the merits of calcium consumed as (a) part of an omnivore (and in some cases, purely carnivore) diet; or perhaps (b) a regime resembling something closer to an herbivore (vegetarian/vegan) diet, it is important to know that you are aiming for your lady to consume a minimum of 1,300mg (milligrams) a day. With vitamin D, you should be targeting 600 IU (international units) a day. Protein guidance varies according to how much your partner weighs, but the general average is about 70 grams a day.

Iron, which is used to make hemoglobin (a protein in the red blood cells that carries oxygen from lungs to the rest of the body), should be consumed in daily quantities of approximately 25-30mg a day. Pregnant women typically require double the amount of iron than women normally need. Hence, it is important as a way to guard against anemia.

This subsection wouldn't be complete without a few considerations around what not to take. Typically, health care professionals warn against taking high-dose multivitamin supplements, fish liver oil supplements, or any supplements containing vitamin A.

I have included this section because despite being a lot to take on, by knowing some of this information, you are better equipped to support your partner and help relieve some of the stress from having to remember all of this stuff. The above guidance represents my finest efforts as an amateur (at best) student of pregnancy nutrition. This is a combination of information provided to me and some that I wish had been provided to me. As always, we suggest that you check any nutritional queries and or actions with your healthcare professional.

Exercise

Exercise during pregnancy can split opinions. To some people who are less knowledgeable and less equipped for pregnancy (i.e. men), there is a preconception that exercise can somehow be dangerous to the unborn child. Generally speaking, your lady can maintain most forms of exercise during pregnancy, but with the guiding principle being that she should not overdo it.

Despite the aches and pains that a woman will begin to experience during pregnancy, exercise is generally considered to help with backaches, bloating and swelling. Similarly it should help the expecting mother with energy levels, while contributing to better sleep and even help you to prepare for labor and birth. It will likely not come as a surprise to hear that the natural endorphins (happy hormones) which are generated via exercise will give her a positive boost and contribute to a cheerful mood. I have discussed how much of a difference this can make.

Generally speaking, low impact exercise methods are favored and recommended. Activities in this category include, walking, stationary cycling, stepping machines and swimming Pregnancy pilates and yoga are great for her body and mind. We further discuss the benefits of meditation in the next chapter, on how you can help your partner through various ups and downs by supporting her mental health.

Your partner should stop exercising and see a healthcare provider if she experiences any chest, abdominal or pelvic pain. Similarly, headaches, dizziness, feeling faint or light-headed should also require a check-up. If your lady notices any increase or decrease in movement from the unborn baby, bleeding and or any discharge of fluid, then they should be checked over as well as any irregular or rapid heartbeat, shortness of breath, muscle weakness and or feeling cold or clammy.

Just to ease your mind, these symptoms do not, by any stretch of the imagination, mean the worst. In many cases, it can be just your partner's body sending her a pace car signal. For example, my wife bled a little after some light exercise and I assumed the absolute worst, only to find out that it is not uncommon and feel somewhat silly (and relieved) for looking like a panic merchant. All in all, however, I would assert that it is better to look like a panic merchant and be safer rather than sorry, as opposed to being Mr. Calm and nonplussed, who then misses a critical opportunity to support their woman and lives to regret it.

Intimacy

Every woman is different during pregnancy. Aside from the raging mix of hormones that will be stampeding through her body and turning many of your partner's usual desires upside down, she may also start to be sensitive to, or self-conscious of, her body image. The result of this can lead to a withdrawal or decrease in her normal sexual appetite and can contribute to anxiety and other mental health hiccups. I am not saying this will definitely happen. Some see a significant rise in sex drive and channel their inner fertile goddess to seek as much pleasure as possible. Others however, prefer to wind it back a little and shift their preferences to being held, gently caressed or some other form of softer physical affection.

Whatever is going on in your partner's inclination for intimacy, it is important that she communicates how she is feeling and what she wants. The same goes for the man, but as she is doing most of the homework on this school project called pregnancy, it is wise if you prioritize her needs accordingly. It is important to pay attention to what she is communicating and to modify your behavior accordingly.

Each relationship and its pair of actors will be unique. But, there is a resounding consensus of opinions across the spectrum of prenatal advice, that intimacy during pregnancy should be encouraged. It is a very sensitive and emotionally potent time and pregnancy professionals will generally suggest that the closer the couple can be together, the better. Furthermore, through the physical connection and sense of lovingness, there are equal mental health benefits. These particularly manifest around body image and giving your lady that inner peace of mind and support that she is indeed still sexy.

In terms of intercourse, often couples will just assume that sex is a nonstarter. This is frequently due to a preconception that you may hurt the baby or the woman. This is typically a myth, or another common male overestimation of their physical (and perhaps phallic) prowess. Intercourse is usually deemed safe, unless directed otherwise by your advising healthcare professional. Yes, your lady may not be overly acrobatic during pregnancy, and you may need to augment your top shelf seduction methods to be more gentle and accommodating, but typically you are able to have as much sex as you both mutually wish to.

Chapter 3

How to Take Care of Her Mentally

During a pregnancy there can be a tendency to focus on the physical aspects of the journey, as it is a very visceral and experiential life event. However, I would argue that the mental health considerations are of equal importance. This opinion is obviously subjective, but my rationale is that the physical experience is largely influenced by the quality of the expecting mother's mental health and further, mental health will be around long after the physical experience has begun to subside. I am by no means a psychologist, but the following items are some general observations and learnings I was fortunate enough to accumulate along the way.

Increase Awareness Towards Her

This may seem obvious, but the first thing to highlight is that an increased level of awareness and vigilance towards your partner during this period is crucial. You may think that the situation's importance will naturally give rise to you simply becoming a 10 out of 10 partner. Maybe you were already at that level and you can only become more awesome and if so, well done. For the little that it is worth, I was in the former category. I simply believed that having a child would remedy a lot of my selfish tendencies and focus my mind on being the best version of myself and as part of that, an awesome support resource for my partner.

Upon reflection, I was either a hopeless optimist in my own capabilities or somewhat deluded. And before you start telling yourself that these descriptions do not fit you, just be aware it is very common to underestimate the level of presence, care and consideration your partner needs during this period. The good thing to remember though, is that it doesn't make you a bad person. It just makes you human. As with many large and important life events, there is a natural human tendency to underestimate the required effort to successfully manage them, combined with a predisposition to overestimate our own preparedness. This plays out time and time again, so even if you are still shaking your head right now, in the least, it may help by prompting some self-reflection.

Being more present, considerate and caring while your partner is experiencing a shifting physical and mental landscape can also be challenging as they start to experience physical discomfort such as nausea, sore breasts, frequent urination and possibly, constipation. These symptoms are common in the first 12 weeks of pregnancy and are often accompanied by their frequent collaborator, the mood swing. We will touch on a few of these ailments later in the First Trimester section.

Understanding the implications of these dynamics at the simplest level requires you to stay alert to problems, frequently monitor whether you need to provide support and assess where you may need to seek third party help.

Due to the rapid changes that a woman undergoes during pregnancy, it is very common to experience fluctuating temperament during pregnancy. The increased mix of hormones that are rushing around her body to help it both prepare for this momentous event and provide all the nutrition and life-support required to grow a human from scratch, is truly one of life's amazing features. With changes in the biochemistry, naturally comes the propensity to experience stress, anxiety and depression. One of the red flags you should be looking out for in this area is persistent anxiety and depression, i.e. where the mood and or sense of wellbeing does not improve over time, or worsens. If your partner is experiencing negative emotions continuously, you will likely need to try and help her to see a healthcare professional.

Depression During Pregnancy (Prenatal)

Depression is a prevalent condition and can be inhibiting during pregnancy. The National Centre for Biotechnology Information refers to studies that show that depression during pregnancy may disrupt fetal growth. Moreover, there is evidence of correlation between a mother's stress levels and low birth weight, premature birth and fetal *hypoxia*, because of lack of oxygen to the unborn child.

However manifested, depression can be disturbing during pregnancy and impede the mother's (and father's) ability to get ready for the imminent delivery of your bundle of joy. Not treating it immediately is dangerous and the longer it goes untreated, the higher the risks attached to it. For some women, depression can also lead to self-destructive behavior around substance abuse and alcohol use, potential weight gain through poor diet and in some cases, a lack of the ability to practice prenatal care.

Fortunately, my wife didn't experience too many low points during her pregnancy journey. That said, I witnessed some of my closest friends wrestle with this specter and it can be incredibly tough. If your partner and or your partner's family have a history of depression, it is likely that she will be more prone to experiencing depression during her pregnancy. However, it is important to note that depression during pregnancy can also occur in women without a clear history of depression. The Mayo Clinic reports that about 7% of pregnant women experience depression throughout their pregnancy.

Typical symptoms may include, continual anxiety about the wellbeing of the unborn child, low self-esteem and feelings of inadequacy around her future parenting skills. There may be an inability to derive pleasure from activities typically found pleasurable, or be unresponsive to reassuring communication and interaction. This can put a strain on your relationship and require some extra empathy and problem solving from you as her partner seeking to care for her. Things get particularly difficult when the expecting mother experiences suicidal ideation and or tendencies. Needless to say, any mix of these symptoms should be assessed, with treatment commenced as soon as humanly possible, regardless of any potential pushback. This is genuinely a scenario where someone's life depends on it.

Other Mental Health Disorders

Naturally, people with all types of challenges and conditions want to be parents and often adults can be exceptional parents in spite of any mental health challenges. That said, for women who have pre-existing conditions such as bipolar disorder, post-traumatic stress disorder, panic attacks, some personality disorders, obsessive compulsive disorder and eating disorders, they will most likely need focused care and support. I want to reiterate that whether your partner has an existing condition, or a history of mental illness, she can, and will likely, still be a brilliant, caring and impactful mother. It may just require a little extra planning and vigilance to ensure both her safety, and that of your unborn daughter or son.

Care and Treatment

As with any health concern during pregnancy, it is important that the mental health issues are dealt with directly and not glossed over or forgotten in the swirling maelstrom of the pregnancy. If your partner is managing any of these conditions or any other mental health hurdle, you should be acutely aware and vigilant for any signs of stress and importantly, work on how you can help. I do appreciate that these are sensitive areas to broach with a loved one, particularly when their body is making hormone molotov cocktails and maybe mischievously playing mental tricks on her, but the guiding north star is to keep your partner and your unborn child safe. You may have to be temporarily unpopular at times to do so.

If your partner is actively managing a mental health condition, then they will most likely discuss and manage the condition with their healthcare provider, with the pregnancy in mind. Where mental health challenges surface during pregnancy, she should get professional help as soon as it is practical. The sooner, the better. At a more personal level, the quicker she starts feeling better, the better it will be for both of you.

Like managing mental health when not pregnant, the typical treatments are likely to be some combination of talking therapy either one on one or via a support group; and or prescription medications. Often frequent support from family and friends can be a potentially less confronting or intrusive alternative to third-party treatment.

It is very important that if your partner is taking some form of mental health prescription medicine, that she checks with a professional before altering the dose. For example, many antidepressants are generally safe to use. That said, equally there are some medicines in this area which can impact a developing baby, so again, please check any considerations with your dedicated health care professional.

Mindfulness, Meditation and Yoga

More frequently in recent decades, pregnant women have found mental health benefits from wellness activities such as mindfulness meditation, deeper forms of meditation and yoga. Mindfulness is considered helpful for the expecting mother to "check in" with herself and pay attention to her body and mind, which are central to the changes she is experiencing. Deeper forms of meditation can add a richer sense of relaxation and mental regeneration. Yoga is excellent as it combines several aspects of a physical workout, which can help with aches and pains, as discussed in the previous chapter. Whichever wellness activity your partner is into should be supported and encouraged, and if she is not, perhaps this life-changing event that is coming down the tracks gives her (and you) the license to experiment and try new things. As a recent yoga skeptic who is now a convert, I can't recommend it enough, and seeing the impact on my wife during her pregnancy, was all the proof I needed.

Depression After the Birth (Postpartum)

We have touched on depression during pregnancy, but this section would not be complete without touching on postpartum depression. Considering the various topics covered, it may come as no surprise that most new mothers will expect some form of mood swings after childbirth. The mix of hormones, emotions, and lack of sleep from the little one developing its nightlife rituals and exacting its demands, can make for a powerful concoction of ups and downs. In the eye of the storm of these downs, things can take on warped dimensions. You may well find yourself wondering how on earth you got here and who in the hell is the crazed person yelling at you? In this scenario, it is likely you may be screaming back with equal voracity, albeit in hushed bursts so as not to wake the baby who has been toying with you both for the last three hours. I slightly digress, but these fluctuating moods are often fondly referred to as the "baby blues."

Postpartum depression, however, is a more extreme and longer lasting form of depression, which can be very hard to experience and manage. It can be equally harrowing for the father to support his partner through such a test. It can be easy to feel powerless to help. The symptoms are similar to those listed above in the prenatal depression section. However, postpartum depression is more severe and may include excessive crying and feelings of hopelessness, worthlessness, futility, shame, and guilt. A woman suffering from this condition may have trouble bonding with her baby, socializing with family and friends, and potentially developing insomnia.

At the most concerning end of the spectrum, she may have thoughts of self-harm and harming the newborn baby, which can compound the sense of guilt, shame, and futility. Needless to say, these symptoms are very troubling and put immense pressure on everyone involved. That said, it is crucial to be aware of the fact that if it goes untreated, it can last for months and possibly much longer. Therefore, such a condition needs focused and ongoing care immediately.

New fathers have been shown to experience postpartum depression too. They may feel anxious, sad, overwhelmed, and experience changes to diet and sleeping. There is a higher risk in men who have historically experienced relationship challenges and or are struggling financially. Later, you will learn how to look after yourself and prepare financially in the following two chapters. But, needless to say you have a responsibility to not only look after your partner, but also yourself. If you are struggling in this area even just a little, or you are experiencing ups and downs which you just can't shake, please reach out and see a mental health professional.

I like to try and end on high notes and so while we have discussed some heavier topics and associated considerations in this chapter, I want to remind us of some positives. It definitely pays to be aware of the spectrum of possible mental health hurdles and associated risks that may need negotiation. But, you can do a lot to help your lady's mental health by just being committed every day. I don't say this to sound trite, rather that this was a lesson I wish I had learned during the first trimester, as opposed to the third one. For example, simple mundane things like doing the dishes, voluntarily cleaning your artistry off the toilet bowl, vacuuming, picking up dinner from the supermarket, and telling her she is still beautiful while she obsesses over her new stretch marks can make all the difference. I firmly believe this and found it to be true during my wife's pregnancy. At the same time, I am not one for unnecessarily rose-tinted glasses or being in denial. If you sense there is a mental health problem brewing or coming to a head, you need to do whatever you can to help her manage it. Point blank, this could be one of the most critical undertakings of your adult life.

<u>Chapter 4</u>

How to Take Care of Yourself

Rightly so, there is a lot of focus on the woman during pregnancy. They are doing most of the work, carrying your child for nine months and then nourishing it for as long as it makes sense after the birth. Just because your partner bears the child, does not mean that the pregnancy isn't happening to, and for, you also.

Deciding to have a child, whether it was long thought out, or a slightly more spontaneous chain of events, can trigger deep emotional and psychological responses. Some of these are pleasant, like excitement, anticipation and the thrill of experiencing everything with your partner. Some may be less enjoyable, like uncertainty, anxiety and fear. As I mentioned earlier, the good news is that all of these emotions, and many more, are completely normal. Furthermore, the more uncomfortable emotions do not mean anything negative or that you are a bad person, just that you are a person. In this chapter, we discuss several ways to look after yourself, be prepared, and ultimately get through this little family-defining odyssey.

Find Role Models

This chapter is short and sweet, because we are men. Men are stoic masters of their emotions. They are bastions of self-belief, resolve and conviction. Men don't need help, a fuss or paragraphs of self-indulgent introspection for comfort. Men are MEN... At least that's what the illusion we like to tell ourselves. To be clear, I am not any type of man that I just described, save for maybe the one who likes illusions. Embarking on my Clueless Dad rite of passage, I needed help. I had fear and uncertainty, it may have been coupled with excitement, but these disagreeable emotions were still there. I had to work hard to manage them and to be better for my wife and future daughter. I also had to work hard to be better for myself. I wasn't prepared to accept a sub-par performance in this area, but I knew it was a tall peak to climb.

While I have been jotting down things in this book that worked for me, there is no denying that I was lucky to receive some great advice from some genuine "men" in my friendship and family circles. These men that I was able to glean various lessons from gave so selflessly and graciously to my cause. They had all been through the fatherhood journey before and had the stories and learnings to share. In my view, they were real MEN, balanced, self-aware, not afraid to be vulnerable, make mistakes, and learn. But, they were also steady, reliable, and supportive as providers for their respective families.

These types of men and countless others who you may have access to in your life are the shortest route to acquiring some fatherhood wisdom ahead of the big day. Yes, there is only so much they or this book can tell you. You have to experience it to properly understand it, but you can do a lot of pre-work by asking the right questions and actively seeking the corresponding answers. In the end, you don't have much to lose. Besides, it is worth remembering that sometimes these types of questions can lead to the shortest routes to examples of what not to do, which can be equally (if not more) valuable than advice on what to do.

Be Mentally Healthy

Like any process or journey of challenging personal growth, it helps to be in the best mental state you can achieve. This isn't some motivational goal hashtag. It is pretty plain common sense. There will be a lot of demands made on you direct and indirectly during the pregnancy, the labor, and the months that follow. While we all wish for an event-free pregnancy, labor, and introduction to parenthood, the truth is any number of hurdles may be presented to you along the way. As such, you should look after yourself, similar to the suggestions made in the sections on looking after her.

Try to get enough sleep, exercise, and practice some form of mental wellness or relaxation. Any form of mindfulness, a deeper form of meditation, or yoga will help you stay balanced. It doesn't even need to be a large commitment. I used both the larger mainstream meditation apps, Headspace and Calm, at different stages during pregnancy and into parenting (I have no relationship with them other than as a customer). I had never meditated before my wife became pregnant. I only started at the recommendation of a friend of mine who swore by it. I have to admit, I was a little skeptical before. It was a foreign concept to me and not something I had been exposed to much through my life. However, I still meditate to this day as often as I can. The impact it had has been seismic, and it has definitely made me a calmer and more grounded parent.

Suppose you are not into those "softer" forms of self-care. In that case, frequent exercise is not only a good idea for your physical wellbeing but also manufacturing some endorphins and knocking out some prospective anxiety. You don't need to be at the level of some 8-packed Instagram influencer who has #nodaysoff. Regular ongoing exercise, whether cardio, strength, or flexibility, can only be positive (provided you don't hurt yourself). For those who are still not convinced, walks in nature, whether in parks, along trails, or on beaches, can also help you unwind and get the blood pumping. We aren't trying to become Iron Man triathletes. We are trying to be the best versions of ourselves for our partner and our unborn child. We owe it to both of them as well as ourselves.

Lastly, in the realm of physical and mental health, men should also be aware of their own needs when it comes to intimacy. While the advice in Chapter 2 regarding intimacy and the recommended action of accommodating your lady as a priority still stands, it is a two-way street. You should be mindful of and comfortable expressing what is important to you. You may start to feel as though the romance is waning with your partner if you do not. It doesn't mean you have to be demanding and or self-centered. Instead, you are gently seeking a way to meet your needs while concurrently striving to meet hers.

This goes much deeper than the physical connection. It is about being on the same page mentally and perhaps even spiritually. While you may not think you will be affected but the experience, you will have a good chance. Therefore, you want to eliminate any feelings of rejection, lacking connection, and or unfulfillment from your partner, whether real or perceived. The stronger your bond is, the more likely you will both get through this test in one piece and happy on the other side. The simplest and most obvious (if not most frequently forgotten way) is via constant open communication.

Journal

I was in two minds whether to discuss daily journaling because it can really split opinion. For those who value it, the act can become a powerful daily habit that can positively influence how a person sets up, executes, and then reviews their day. It is like mentally flossing or brushing your teeth daily. When done regularly, you just mentally minty fresh and a little more mentally prepared. It can seem like a lofty chore done by snowflakes too worried about thoughts and feelings for those who don't value it.

I think the common misconception is that to journal well, you need to have a point of view, be brilliant at prose, or say something personal that someone might find one day and make the writer feel embarrassed. Equally, people may feel like it is pointless, that there are better things to do and that the process of reviewing one's thoughts and behaviors can be confronting. This is particularly the case when we are faced with certain things about ourselves that may be uncomfortable.

You don't need to be Mark Twain to journal well. The process is much more of a way to tidy up the noise in our heads, get clear on the important things, and throw away those that aren't. I find five to ten minutes of journaling in the morning helps me declutter the noise that my mind has a habit of creating.

Sometimes I just recount what I have been doing in my morning routine or something I have been reading. During both pregnancies that I have been a part-owner in, I have journaled to organize my thoughts, manage my concerns, and identify the priority areas. A huge beneficial byproduct of this is that I have a record of the processes that led to my most favorite humans' birth.

Be Prepared

We have touched on being prepared in several areas already. However, it is worth reiterating it again. While pregnancies have a pretty decent normal distribution in terms of how they unfold, they do also have an endless number of potential variables. As you are undertaking a monumental task that will come with some sense of uncertainty, perhaps at times anxiety, the best antidote is preparedness. You will not be able to prepare for every possible eventuality, but you can cover a lot with a little work.

Given the ubiquity of the internet and the fact that we and our ancestors have been giving birth for millions of years, you can generally find answers to most questions you will have on the topic. There is a lot of decent written content, several mobile apps and some key websites, that we suggest you spend some time on when upskilling on the roles and responsibilities of taking the First-time Dad job.

Many couples will naturally attend antenatal classes to both to acquire knowledge, but also to support your lady. While Hollywood has somewhat incorrectly shaped many of our preconceptions around these antenatal classes, they remain one of the best ways to learn about becoming a parent while getting an in-depth look at the primary considerations, key milestones, and risk areas throughout the pregnancy. The thought of learning birthing plans with complete strangers may fill you with dread, but it is necessary, and in the end, you will find it highly valuable.

Finally, it is worth touching on the use of counseling to be prepared and manage any niggling mental health concerns you may have. This is a topic that many men avoid discussing. Ever since we are babies, we have teachers, coaches, and mentors. It is often lost on me why we don't have them for the most important areas of our lives unless it is in a crisis. Remember the good old airline warning, "you should fit your own oxygen mask before you fit anyone else's." It is good advice. It may be repetitive and sometimes downright irritating, but this is often a hallmark of good advice. As such, the premise should be heeded. How can you help your loved ones if you haven't helped yourself first? It is a necessary undertaking and one that can significantly reduce unnecessary stress.

Chapter 5

How to Prepare Financially

This is an area where even the most successful and financially stable prospective fathers can catch some jitters. You will have heard the timeless and frequently used mantra that says, 'there is no perfect time to have a baby." Well, I am here to wholeheartedly agree. I never really thought about being a father growing up, and so I can't really claim that I had a clear vision for it. That said, I intuitively expect to be at least a homeowner (no matter how modest), not to be thousands of dollars in debt with some cash in the bank, and ideally, not about pursuing a postgraduate degree. I was firmly at sea with these waves of economic and personal growth pressures battering away at my vessel. I was definitely on board to start a family with my wife. But my lack of progress, when compared to my expectations, did cause me some grief. This chapter contains some practical advice to ease the strain and get your head in the financial preparation game.

If you are reading this from outside the US, some of the figures provided below may not be completely relevant, but the considerations around how to optimize costs will be, so I would gently suggest you persevere if you can find it within you.

Planning, Budgeting and Workarounds for a Newborn

Your newborn will not actually cost as much as you think early on. Yes, some birthing costs can hurt the wallet depending on which country you live in. And yes, there are some ubiquitous costs. These being namely the crib; the pram (later the stroller); a collection of newborn paraphernalia for feeding, sleeping, bathing; clothes; and potentially, decorating the new addition's room. However, a newborn's operating costs are pretty low for the first three to six months. This is because they, and as a result, you, don't do that much. They rely on their mother for milk, sleep a lot, and really just going through diapers and the odd bath.

Having eased you in with a little short-term hope, we can start to cover less exciting areas to work on to get yourself in a decent financial state ahead of delivery time. I mentioned several one-time setup purchases you will likely need to make in the paragraph above. Still, you will also need to start to estimate and budget for your ongoing weekly expenses. While diapers are one of the most common expenses people think of, you should go broad to make sure sure you don't have any nasty surprises down the line. For example, you may have been expecting your baby to be costing $200 an extra week, and for some reason, it is $250 per week.

Like anything to do with cash outflows, the more you plan, the more likely it will be accurate. It is imperative that you understand all the setup costs and then monthly or weekly running costs. Once you have a full picture of the demands, it is possible to take steps to offset these expenses, should you be so minded. For example, we bought a second hand, top tier pram for our little angel off eBay and bulk bought diapers to keep costs down. We then managed to plan ahead to secure a bulk discount when we purchased the baby's crib and stand, mattress, linen, sleep monitor, changing table, and rocking chair, all from the same supplier.

We weren't flush with cash at the time. But, we were earning adequate salaries and could have stretched to a brand new pram's price. However, we started to think of:

How short the time will be that our child will actually use the pram (likely to grow out of it in less than six months).

The abundance of pre-loved baby equipment in the world and the corresponding impact this has on lowering prices.

What else we could do with the savings made on such a purchase.

As a result, we came to the conclusion that it just didn't make sense to pay thousands of dollars for something you could get clean, lightly used, and just as good, for a couple of hundred dollars. Yes, we felt a little conflicted because we wanted everything "brand new" for our little princess, but at the same time, we deemed this point of contention as a primarily superficial concern. I am in no way against spending whatever you wish on your child. This is your right, and no one should tell you otherwise. All I am saying is that if you need, or wish, to be slightly more frugal, there are generally ways to accomplish it.

Healthcare Costs

Depending on where you live, having a baby can be expensive. In some countries like the United Kingdom, births are entirely covered by the National Health Service, unless the parents choose to go through health insurance and use private facilities. Conversely, it will be no surprise for US readers that the US is one of the most expensive places to have a baby, along with Japan. In 2019, Business Insider reported on statistics provided by FAIR Health, the US average cost to have a baby was $10,808, provided that it was a normal vaginal birth. Using similar data, website parents.com reported that on average, a Cesarean-section ('C-section') birth costs $16,106. By comparison, "normal" deliveries cost $3,195, and C-sections cost $5,980 in Canada.

As a start, to give an indication of the variation in birthing costs across the US, we look at data that FAIR Health provided Business Insider comprising the costs of individual states. Alabama is the cheapest state to have a baby in, with a vaginal birth costing $5,230.46 and a C-section costing $8,221.42, both with insurance. This is compared to $9,516.86 for a vaginal birth and $13,589.75 for a C-section, both without insurance. Alaska is the most expensive state, with $11,609.95 for a vaginal birth and $16,797.29 for a C-section, both with insurance. This compares to $20,243.38 and $28,617.34, respectively, without insurance. There is a vast collection of variations within these ranges.

For low to middle-income families, these figures can be challenging to process. The costs are mitigated to some degree by insurance, but they remain relatively quite high when compared to the average wage bands. If you are fortunate to ease the burden through insurance, make sure to plan for the process and amend yours or your partner's insurance policy accordingly to cover the pregnancy. It can be challenging to do this later down the road.

When considering healthcare costs, you should ensure you have adequately considered and budgeted for prenatal care. These are all the check-ups, scans, and other pregnancy-related appointments your partner will need to attend leading up to the birth. Parents are often so focused on the cost of the delivery itself. They neglect to properly budget for the ongoing appointments and other fees required at different times during the trimesters. While estimating these, don't forget to include the prenatal and parenting classes that can be done online or in community groups of couples expecting around the same time. These are not always technically considered healthcare costs, but they form part of the prenatal expenses you will need to build into your budget and planning.

Postnatal Budgeting

Having recovered from the discomfort of your early budgeting activities and understanding the full extent of the potential financial burden of the birth, it is then worth turning your attention to your longer-term plan. Asking parents how much a child costs to raise really is a "how long is a piece of string" question. It depends on the country, location within that country, urban versus rural living, income bands, socio-economic views, and the parents' own perception of the value of education, to name a few. While some of these drivers are macro-level influences, many of them are individual and deeply personal.

To provide you with some ballpark reference figures, the USDA estimates that, on average, a child will cost $233,610 from birth until they turn 17. This figure is reflected in a two-parent, two children, middle-income family. From birth until the child is two years old, the USDA suggests that the annual average is $12,680. This, however, increases steadily, reaching $13,180 by age nine and $13,900 by the time they are later stage teenagers leading up to 17.

Education is the classic hallmark focus in this area of budgeting. In the modern age, the "college fund" has become the phantom second mortgage that parents simply take on as a necessity to give their children the best possible start. As touched on above, your perception and assessment of an education's value significantly impact your appetite to create a college fund. The same can be said regarding your decisions around private versus public education, homeschooling versus group classes, and going away to college compared to going straight into the workforce.

Given the proliferation of the internet in recent decades, current workplace trends toward remote working, and the shifting skillsets towards technology, there is likely to be significant disruption to the preconceptions around higher education that we had growing up. For example, there is already a growing argument that it makes little sense for your child to incur huge student debts to attend college when they can likely learn everything they need online and at a fraction of the cost. This viewpoint is likely to increase with technologically-focused jobs, like coding, data analytics, and other quantitative disciplines, which can be delivered online, becoming dramatically more in demand. The result of which likely diminishes the argument for expensive location-based tuition further.

To be clear, I am not saying there will no longer be the need for universities and or going away to college. This stage in a young person's life has long been considered a rite of passage, and I certainly remember those years fondly. However, I am saying that there are fundamental changes underway in how society perceives education, how it is delivered, and the cost to acquire it. These changes will likely impact our own views and the perspectives of our children. These changes can affect the levels to which we are either willing to or deem it necessary to budget for our children's educational futures.

A Rainy Day Fund

I would posit that most adults are familiar with the concept of a rainy day fund. This being, a pot of money put away for emergencies or if anything goes wrong. They can be challenging to commit to if you are particularly efficient at matching your income with your expenditure and find it quite hard to save money. I should admit that the concept of a rainy day fund is difficult for me to adhere to. Currently, I know what they are, and I know I should have one, but I would be equally hypocritical and dishonest if I told you to create one without coming clean that I have not always been successful in this area. This is mainly because creating a rainy day fund is like another insurance policy that you aren't forced to take, but that can make all the difference. You know they are essential, but the fact that they are not mandatory means that when push comes to shove, they require self-discipline and a little sacrifice. By nature, these two qualities can provide a little discomfort. Regardless of the discomfort they can cause, you don't need to be a genius to know that this type of fallback resource when things get bad is good common sense and provides a layer of security to you and your family.

Early on, I committed and started to build a rainy day fund. It was like pulling teeth, but after I picked up some momentum, I did start to enjoy it. I began to derive pleasure from knowing I had it, that I had exhibited some self-control and discipline. However, more recently, my wife and I decided to use our rainy day fund to move internationally with our children. We justified it because we could give our children a better quality of life at the intended destination. Now the merit of that decision is subjective, but we were only able to make that decision because… you guessed it, we actually had a rainy day fund.

After a series of very trialing career circumstances, we made that decision which led to me resigning from work and needing to make some quick, wholesale changes. This, combined with a deep desire to provide our children's best possible life, was our joint motivation. Now, I realize that resigning may not constitute something going bad or a particular emergency in certain people's eyes. I can respect that, but I would also suggest that all life challenges are relative, and what is one person's emergency may, in fact, not be another's. The purpose of this little anecdote is not to invite your judgment on what constitutes an emergency for me, but rather to prompt you to think about what would constitute one for you. Having done that thought experiment, I also wanted to highlight that a rainy day fund, while a total chore to put together, provided me with the flexibility to make life choices for my family on my own terms. I was able to leave an employment situation that was negatively impacting my life, my health, and my ability to be a functional husband and father. If I was still stuck there, there is no telling how much worse things could have got.

Wouldn't you like to have that level of flexibility and optionality in your life? If so, start a rainy day fund. It doesn't matter how modest it is. The key is to build the financial muscle of doing it. You never know when you may need it, but all you know for sure is that one day, you will need it.

Longer Term Considerations

There is no doubt that several of the things mentioned above require commitment and planning. However, you mustn't focus on short to medium-term considerations at the expense of long-term planning and financial security. To close out this chapter, I touch on some of the more "grown-up" elements of how to prepare financially.

First of all, do not stop contributing to your long-term financial assets, whether they include life insurance, pension, or other types of retirement plan. Secondly, make sure that you create or update a will. This may seem a low priority as we all believe we are going to live forever. But, just in case that expectation proves to be incorrect, it doesn't hurt to have one. Thirdly, make sure you add any additional beneficiaries to your insurance, retirement plans, or any other form of financial asset you are building for your family's future. It is tempting to think that if something does happen to us, our partners will look after things. You may be right, but there is no harm in preparing for all potential scenarios, and further, it doesn't hurt to gently push your lady to do the same.

In the end, a little bit of planning now will significantly outweigh the cost of being unprepared in most of the cases above. Regardless of how low the likelihood is, you can reduce a lot of extra stress and or pressure on your family in the event of an unforeseen crisis or tragedy by taking some small steps to shore up their future.

Chapter 6

The First Trimester

The beginning of the first trimester is a sneaky time. Your partner will not necessarily be pregnant in the first couple of weeks of your specified pregnancy period. As previously mentioned, this can mean that sometimes the woman does not know she is pregnant until somewhere between the fourth and sixth week, or even longer in some cases. If you have been trying for a long time with limited success or you have just started, it can really catch you by surprise. Continuing with the theme that each pregnancy is unique, the way your lady's body can respond can be anywhere on the spectrum from glowing invincibility to aches, discomfort, and nausea. Some people experience an irritating blend of these extremes and a mix of other physical symptoms. Needless to say, there are myriad biological wonders afoot during this time. The little fertilized egg is multiplying and replicating cells at a rapid pace. While many changes are invisible other changes, naturally, some of the more visible changes will start to fill you and your partner with excitement. The following contents of this chapter set out some things to look out for and consider and some tips to make the process easier.

Depending on who you speak to, there are differing views on the exact number of weeks within the three trimesters. For the avoidance of any doubt, we use the pregnancy calendar provided by John Hopkins Medicine. As such, we discuss the first trimester from week 1 to week 12.

Due Date Calculator

Get yourself a due date calculator. These are typically mobile apps or web portals that you and your partner can track your baby's development. This may seem trivial, but it's not. You will be amazed at your little guy or girl's growth and development in such a short time. As an aside, these digital helpers can also provide additional guidance and support to help with any emotional, physical, and or mental hurdles the woman needs to navigate. They are an excellent little resource to make the process go more smoothly.

Conception & Implantation

Given that conception will typically occur around two weeks after your partner's prior period began. Doctors and or health care professionals will allocate the 40 week gestation period from that date. Needless to say, there is not a lot to be aware of at the beginning.

Around week three, the sperm and the egg will connect in one of your partner's fallopian tubes. This creates a single cell called a zygote. Sometimes two eggs are released and fertilized, or a fertilized egg splits into two, and there become several zygotes. While we don't need to go into a full biology lesson, it is worth noting that the zygote usually has 46 chromosomes, 23 from each parent. I found that interesting once I understood how early this occurs as these chromosomes help decide whether you are having a boy or girl. After the zygote is fertilized, it then travels back down the fallopian tube to the uterus while concurrently splitting into multiple cells.

By week 4, the group of cells is dividing rapidly and is now known as a blastocyst. This ball of cells has also started to tunnel into the uterus lining and implant itself. The cells in the middle of the blastocyst will become the embryo soon after. The outer group of the blastocyst cells will become the placenta, which provides much of the nutrition to the baby during the gestation period.

Hello Embryo

After the implantation (around week 5), there is an increase in the levels of the Human Chorionic

Gonadotropin hormone (hCG) produced by the blastocyst. Interestingly hCG can be detected as early as one week after fertilization and forms the basis for most over-the-counter pregnancy tests. In fact, the woman's hCG levels every two to three days as the embryo continues to develop, but the levels peak around week six. The hCG levels will start to decrease after this point, and interestingly after the placenta has completed forming, the assistance of hCG to support the ovaries is no longer required. Following this spike in hCG, the ovaries are given the nod to stop producing eggs and go to work, producing more estrogen and progesterone. These increased levels of hormones are what also signals a halt to the woman's period cycles.

By this stage, the embryo is made up of three layers: the ectoderm, the mesoderm, and the endoderm. The ectoderm is the top layer and will develop into the baby's outermost layer of skin, nails, the eye's lens, inner ears, nasal cavity, mouth, tooth enamel, and the central and peripheral nervous systems, to name a few. The mesoderm, the middle layer, will develop into your little one's heart and circulatory system, kidneys, reproductive system, bones, muscles, and ligaments. The endoderm forms the inner layer of cells and will develop into the baby's intestines, liver, pancreas, and lungs.

With all the body parts starting to come together, growth takes off in week six. Being only four weeks since conception, there is a tube along the baby's back that begins to close. This is called the neural tube, and the baby's brain and spinal will develop from this part of the embryo. There are little bumps where the arms will grow that start to protrude. Simultaneously, some of the structures required to house the eyes and ears will be forming, as will be the heart's early stages and other vital organs.

It was pretty mind-blowing for me to learn that the baby's heart can start beating around 22 days after conception. It just seemed so quickly for such a vital and complex organ to start working away, even if not fully formed yet. You will typically be able to hear the heartbeat around week 12, which is why waiting to tell anyone outside the two of you is often recommended until after this point. However, it may be possible to pick up a heartbeat as early as around weeks six to eight.

Baby's Burst of Physical Development

One of the great things that makes the calculators fun is the ability to track the progress that your little one is making weekly and sometimes even daily. After around week six, the more recognizable features and bursts of development start to occur at a level that we as adults can relate to. In week seven, your baby's features begin to become visible, while the brain, head, and face continue to grow. Little indents and ridges start to signal where the fully formed nose and eyes will one day be. The lower limbs begin to show themselves as well.

By week eight, the baby's fingers have started to develop out of the top limbs. Bearing in mind, this is only really six weeks since conception, the rate of growth has been extraordinary. The lower limbs look like small flippers. Small bumps have emerged around the head, which will develop into ears, and the area where the eyes will develop becomes more defined and pronounced. More of the facial features have taken on a more structured form, particularly with the nose and top lip having developed. On average, the baby is coming up to about 0.63 inches and weighs around 0.04 ounces.

By week nine, your baby is proudly showing off his or her new sets of elbows. They may not be complete yet, but they are there, just as there is an accompanying set of toes starting to show themselves. Your little one has also started to exhibit their eyelids. On average, by week nine, your baby is now around 0.9 inches and weighing 0.07 ounces. This is around the size of a penny, which feels very small. This is *circa* 42% increase in size and nearly doubling in weight, which is impressive for your little girl or guy.

The head has continued to grow throughout these early stages, and by week ten, it has taken on more of a rounded skull shape, transitioning from the blob shape that it started as. At this stage, a rather cute thing to know is that the baby can start to bend its elbows. Also, the fingers and toes begin to lose their webbing and become more distinct individual structures. The eyelids and external ears continue to grow into their own, and the umbilical cord is readily visible. It is important to note that leading up to week 11, your baby's head is still over half the baby's length, which will have increased to around 1.22 inches. At this stage, the embryo is weighing about 0.14 ounces.

Leveling Up from Embryo to Fetus

Welcome to week 11 (week 9 since conception), and your baby graduates from elementary school to middle school. Congratulations! Your little one is now considered a fetus. At this point, your baby's body is about to start making bursts of growth to catch up with the head. During this stage, the face is taking on more features with the eyes separating towards their final resting places. The eyelids are fused together, bumps where the teeth will eventually appear to start to make their presence seen. Your baby's genitals start to develop towards the end of this week, and it is wild to imagine that this little entity's red blood cells have started to congregate in the early stages of the liver.

Week 12 marks the end of the first trimester and a significant milestone. Your little one has achieved remarkable progress. Having moved from the darkness of non-existence to conception only 10 weeks earlier, bones, muscles, and working organs began. In addition, your little one's cranium and face have significantly developed, with early-stage eyes, ears, nose, and mouth. Around 12 weeks, your baby has started to grow fingernails, and their intestines are embedded in the abdomen. Mother nature is truly undefeated!

By week 12, your little person is over 2 inches in length and weighing in at a massive 0.5 ounces. He or she will be starting to make their presence felt and getting ready for the second trimester. Well done on getting this far, and hopefully, you have found it enjoyable, humbling, and educational.

Your Lady's Body

While tracking your little one's progress can be exciting and enlightening, let's not forget that your partner will be experiencing any number of side effects. While you can't necessarily take any of these off her plate, you can be aware of them and ease any discomfort symptoms. We covered several items to be mindful of during the chapter on How to Take Care of Her Physically. Still, a few other ailments or physical conditions may or may not reveal themselves during this period.

Not long after conception, the burst of hormones and changes in the body to stimulate and manage the embryo's development can make your lady's breasts swollen and sore. This typically mirrors the changes in the milk production elements of your lady's breasts getting ready to feed your baby. This is definitely not something you can help with. However, it is worth being aware that she may need to go up a bra size or retire some of the fancier bras for some months in exchange for more comfortable and functional support bras. This is likely to be the case until she is no longer nursing the baby.

Progesterone is a powerful and critical hormone during pregnancy, particularly early on. But, it can be a pesky additive for your lady's body. While potentially playing judo with her breasts, it can also lead to heartburn. This is because progesterone has a muscle-relaxing effect. This muscle relaxation also impacts the esophagus, which usually keeps food and stomach acids down in the belly. With a relaxed gateway to the stomach, so to speak, this allows for acid reflux, or more commonly, heartburn. It is typically recommended that the woman eat smaller meals, more often during the day. It is also suggested that the woman should not lie down immediately after eating, and she should swerve particularly acidic, spicy, and or greasy foods.

Bleeding during pregnancy can be a distressing symptom for obvious reasons. The good thing is it is often not as bad as it may seem. It is worth noting that statistics suggest that approx. 25% of women will experience slight bleeding during the first trimester.

As well-adjusted men, we never shy away from understanding some of the less glamorous elements of pregnancy and the journey our ladies are on. As part of this, it is worth noting that the hormone progesterone discussed earlier in this chapter can slow down digestion. This results in making food move more slowly through the woman's intestines, which, when combined with the increased iron intake from her prenatal supplement regime, results in uncomfortable constipation and gas. Helping her to keep her fluids up and increase fiber intake will help offset this. In addition, making sure there is a level of physical activity can help "get things moving," instead of being too sedentary.

Another potentially less flattering, but completely natural byproduct of the early stages of pregnancy is the presence of discharge. It is perfectly normal to see a milky, translucent discharge released from the vagina early on in the pregnancy. If your partner experienced this, your healthcare professional will, apart from reassuring your lady that this is normal, recommend that your partner wears a panty liner. They will firmly not recommend using a tampon, to eliminate any risk of introducing any bacteria to the vagina.

This section is designed to help you be prepared, reduce uncertainty, and have a decent understanding of some small speed bumps that could expose themselves along the way. I include various examples of symptoms, causes, and potential mitigants. However, I am in no way making light of any potential health risks, and as always, if you or your partner are unsure or feeling exposed at any time, the best bet is always to see a healthcare professional. In the event of significant dizziness, abdominal pain, bleeding, and or rapid weight loss or weight gain, your partner should see a doctor as soon as possible.

Doctor's Appointments

In today's day and age, most people know to see a doctor as soon as they think they are pregnant. This type of care leading up to the pregnancy referred to as prenatal care, is not a one-size-fits-all structure. Prenatal care can be effectively delivered by any combination of a midwife, family GP, obstetrician, and prenatal group, but it helps to know when and where to seek help.

The first visit will usually comprise an assessment of the woman's medical history. This may include gynecological history, family medical history, any vulnerability of toxic substances, information on prescription medications being used, lifestyle choices around caffeine, tobacco, and alcohol intake. This visit will involve a physical with likely blood tests to make sure everything is healthy and provide your lady with a target due date based upon the timing of the last period and other symptoms.

Following this initial meeting, it is typically recommended that the woman sees a healthcare professional every four weeks or so through the first two trimesters. This then shortens to closer to two weeks through the third trimester. Then likely once a week in the four weeks leading up to the birth.

Apart from the first appointment following determining that the woman is pregnant, any other follow-ups deemed necessary, the next major appointment to be aware of is the week 12 ultrasound scan to ensure that the baby is developing well. In reality, this scan may happen after week eight. This helps give a clearer picture of how long the woman has been pregnant and tighten the expected due date prediction. After this scan, the expecting parents (assuming you both can attend) will be given their first image of their little one on the road to being born.

A common misconception is that at 12 weeks, you will be able to tell the gender of the baby. While the genitals have been developing, it is still too early to know if it is a boy or a girl, should you be motivated to find out. Some people do find out, and some prefer to wait for the surprise at birth. There is no right or wrong approach, and it comes down to the couple's preference. Naturally, there is more on this in the next chapter.

Chapter 7

The Second Trimester

After the somewhat miraculous events that get this whole show on the road, the second trimester is really where the development of your little one shifts gears and makes serious leaps and bounds. The first trimester was more about things happening rapidly, but that may not have been visible to the naked eye. The second trimester definitely brings home how real this experience is. Your lady will start to show tangible physical changes, but this trimester is typically the most physically enjoyable for your partner. The first trimester can hit your lady (and her hormones) like a ton of bricks, while the third trimester can be very uncomfortable as your baby reaches maximum size. For this middle act, I would suggest you chill as much as you can and enjoy the proverbial calm before the storm.

This period of the pregnancy goes from week 13 to week 26. As the baby's proportional rate of growth slows during the second trimester, we move to providing length and weight update on a bi-weekly basis during this chapter.

Baby Keeps on Developing

Week 13 marks your little one's move from elementary to middle school in terms of his or her gestation period. This period is physically notable as the baby's intestines move from within the umbilical cord, where they have been developing, to the abdomen where they will stay. While this little show of independence by the baby is adorable, they aren't quite ready to do everything on their own from a digestive perspective just yet. Your partner's placenta will continue to grow along with the fetus to nourish the child with oxygen and nutrients and get rid of any waste.

At the same time, the little bones that have been developing as arms and legs continue to become more detailed, and the baby may even be able to get the early beginnings of their thumb into their mouth. As previously mentioned, around this time, the heartbeat is more readily detectable.

By week 14, some very fine colorless hair may have developed on your baby's face and will spread across most of their body before shedding just prior to the birth. This hair is called lanugo, and while it may stay with the baby after birth, it will usually be gone by the time the baby is 4 months old, at the very latest. By this time, the baby's genitals are approaching being fully formed, but they may still be a bit elusive to distinguish clearly on a scan.

I was blissfully unaware that around this time, the baby actually takes small sips of amniotic fluid. It is ingested into their stomach, travels through their kidneys, and is excreted as urine. I naively thought that amniotic fluid was purely mother nature's answer to airbags and kept the little one safe from bumps. While It does that part, it also provides hydration and nutrients. We provide more information on amniotic fluid and its role in the overall pregnancy later in the chapter.

It is hard to fathom that your baby has grown from approximately 1 gram of mass to around 43 grams of mass in just a few weeks. Your baby will be weighing on average around 1.5 ounces and is somewhere just under 3.4 inches in length.

Around week 15, it is thought that your baby may start to sense light from outside the mother's stomach, the rhythmic beat of your partner's heart, and potentially muffled sounds from the goings-on a world away outside of the womb. In addition to the delicate hair developing on your baby's body, his or her eyebrows and head hair continue to develop.

The baby's bones and muscles continue to evolve, and movements become more frequent, feeling like little flutters of activity. The little one's ears are nearly in their permanent position, having moved up the side of the head from where they started. Around this time, the baby may start to get hiccups occasionally, which flitter in your partner's abdomen.

Week 16 should be building on the movement that the baby has been getting active in since starting the second trimester. That said, it will not be unusual for your partner to not have felt anything by this stage, so don't worry if this is the case. Some women feel movement early and others do later. It is typically only after around week 24, that you should see a healthcare professional in the event your partner hasn't felt the baby move yet.

Meanwhile, at this stage, the baby is starting to be able to make early-stage facial expressions. They begin to be able to squint and frown, but without any muscular control. Their central nervous system continues to mature, and they can hold their head up a little.

The growth spurt continues, with the length from crown to rump on average reaching around 4.6 inches. Your little one will, on average, weigh approximately 3.53 ounces as the weight continues its acceleration.

Around week 17, your baby is starting to be able to move their eyes (although everything is firmly closed up in that area). If you could actually see them, the eyebrows are making their presence known, and rather cutely, the eyelashes are developing.

While the baby has been growing, so has its partner in crime, the placenta. It has thousands of blood vessels acting like the baby's on-demand nutrient and oxygen and delivery system. Not only does it sustain and nurture the baby's development, but it is also a pretty efficient waste disposal unit for the baby.

It is pretty mind-blowing to think of your baby having its own unique fingerprint at this stage, but it does. Around this time, there is an inflection point where the body starts to develop and build out so that the head no longer represents the bulk of this important little package. It's been 15 weeks since being conceived, and your little one is powering through this transformation.

By 18 weeks, the baby's sensory systems continue to evolve and strengthen. Their ears are picking up all kinds of noise from inside their mother. This is because the bones and developing cartilage of the ear are maturing in conjunction with the brain's nerves. Around this time, some mothers report that they feel movement that correlates to loud music from outside the womb.

Coincidentally, the baby's ears have reached their final resting position. To the untrained eye (which mine definitely was), it appeared serene and peaceful for the baby to be floating around in a warm nourishing sac of fluid. However, it is filled with loud noises from the mother's heartbeat, breathing, and the loud rushing of blood as it travels around the busy circulation subway system to the placenta and umbilical cord.

At the same time, your little one's eyes are coming into their own. Your baby may even be able to sense light from the bright beams of a torch, or bright light held up to the side of the mother's tummy. Isn't that crazy?

Around this time, on average, the baby's length has reached around 5.6 inches, and its weight will have nearly doubled in two weeks to 6.70 ounces.

Coming through week 19, your baby has started to develop brown fat for insulation after birth. Brown fat will typically make up 5% of the newborn's body weight. This type of fat's primary function is to guard against hypothermia. Hence it will keep the baby warm after birth, as it gets used to life outside. Interestingly, brown fat is found in high levels in hibernating mammals as well, as it is employed during their long periods of sleep through the winter.

Besides making some progress on building out some chubbiness, your little one has also been working on their skincare routine. By this time, their whole body should be covered in a thick greasy white coating called vernix caseosa. It acts like a human form of lanolin, preventing the skin from being chafed. It also protects the baby from any skin damage from being permanently submerged in amniotic fluid and guards against infections.

Week 20 heralds the renowned "20-week scan", which is also referred to as the anomaly scan. It can happen as early as week 18. This scan checks on the baby's growth, helps identify any visible problems or irregular measurements and makes sure the placenta is in good health and where it should be.

Importantly, this scan also provides the opportunity to determine the gender of the baby, which can really split opinion. The 20-week scan has become a bit of a milestone, but it is also worth noting that some eagle-eyed ultrasound technicians will be able to tell you the sex as early as 16 weeks. As an aside, it is worth highlighting that there are different methods to find out the gender of the baby much earlier than 20 weeks, for those who can't wait or where there is a specific need to do so. In reality, some earlier DNA and blood tests can be used from around 10 weeks, but these are typically less common than waiting for the ultrasound.

I must admit that I am a glutton for instant gratification and always ruin my own surprises. In addition, psychologically, I also needed to start getting my head in the game for our impending delivery and needed every little bit of help and preparation time I could find. As a result, we found out the sex of our daughter. I know different people have different beliefs, opinions, and frames of reference. I am certainly not advocating one way or the other. Ultimately it will be up to you and your partner to decide what is best for you regarding this simple but potentially life-changing piece of information.

20 weeks also marks the halfway point for a 40-week gestation period. By this point in the journey, the baby's length has reached around 6.5 inches on average from crown to rump, and its weight will have gone over 10.5 ounces.

By week 21, the baby's bone marrow areas have matured enough to start to help with blood cell production. Until this time, your baby has been relying on its liver and spleen to manufacture new blood cells. This is a sign of things to come. Through the third trimester, the bone marrow will become the major production area for blood cells. It is suggested that the spleen will typically cease producing blood cells by week 30, and the liver stops within a few weeks of the birth. That is a little fun fact you will undoubtedly get to use at a trivia night one day.

Physically, the baby is still growing across all areas, with the head hair and eyebrows becoming more established and transitioning from colorless to containing pigment. The lanugo and vernix caseosa also continue to develop all over the baby.

Week 22 marks a rather cute stage of development of your baby's taste senses. The taste buds have started to develop on the tongue and linked up to the brain via nerve endings. In the beginning, these forming nerve endings manifest themselves by being sensitive to touch. As a result, it will be typical for your baby to start sucking their tiny thumbs and or stroking their own face and other body parts. It must be quite a trip to experience that for the first time. Imagine your barely formed sensations of touch sending little touch sensory signals to your brand-new brain for processing after only 20 weeks since conception.

In other areas of your little one's body, his or her lungs are still forming, and while they won't get a dress rehearsal to work on their own before the birth, the baby starts to practice the movements ahead of the day they start breathing on their own. Until then, the placenta is busy delivering all the oxygen necessary to keep the baby developing, healthy, and safe.

If you are having a boy, his testes have begun to drop into position from where they started in the abdomen. If you are having a girl, the ovaries and uterus have reached their final resting place, and the vagina is finishing forming.

After week 20, as the baby has grown significantly, it is typical to start measuring the baby's length from crown to heel (as opposed to from crown to rump for the first half of the pregnancy). By week 22, the baby will measure an average of around 10.9 inches and continues to put on weight reaching over 12.5 ounces.

Coming into week 23, the baby is still very wrinkly despite the build-up of the brown fat. Your partner may start to feel more lively movement as the baby's muscles across its body start to fire up and become more regular. The little flutters that started to vibrate in your lady's tummy from early movement and hiccups have now leveled up to judo kicks and little punches. This will naturally increase as the baby becomes larger, stronger, and more coordinated. Your partner will also start to recognize patterns in the baby's movements during certain activities or at specific times of the day.

Building on the movement described in the recent weeks, by week 24 your lady may have started to recognize the baby's sleeping patterns and being awake. She may find your little one has no respect for her body clock and is yet to adhere to any form of circadian rhythm. In addition, the baby's inner ear, which manages and regulates its early sense of balance, has matured enough that the baby might be able to sense whether it is upside down or not. This increased sense of positioning by the baby itself also contributes to the movement as it starts to experiment with fixing its position to accommodate being the right way up (which is not always straightforward when you are floating around in another human's tummy).

By week 24, on average, the baby's length has reached around 11.8 inches, and its weight will have broken into measurement by pounds, coming in approximately 1.32 pounds.

By week 25, the baby's core organs, respiratory system, and digestive systems are formed but are still maturing. The strength and complexity of their hearing continue to develop and mature as well.

The baby is also taking on amniotic fluid and passing it as urine.

Around this time, I received another mind-bending piece of intel. I learned that in the unlikely event, the baby needed to be birthed early, the little one would at least have a chance of survival at this point. Healthcare professionals refer to this as the fetus being "viable." He or she would need intensive support and care and would be susceptible to health complications, but it did provide me with a certain sense of relief to know my daughter had made it this far.

Week 26 marks the end of the second trimester and another glorious milestone. Your baby will likely close out this achievement by showing off some skills. Around this time, their eyelids start opening and blinking after having had their eyes firmly closed since conception. The color of your baby's eyes at birth will depend on ethnicity, with some babies will be born with brown or dark eyes. Others will be born with blue or gray-blue eyes.

As the sun sets on this magical trimester, on average, the baby's length (from crown to heel) has reached around 14 inches, and its weight will be around 1.7 pounds. This is a pretty remarkable level from entering this trimester at 2.91 inches from crown to rump and weighing 0.81 ounces. Talk about growth spurt, this is nothing short of spectacular!

The Amniotic Fluid

As the amniotic fluid starts to play an increasingly important supporting role in this second act of the pregnancy, I have included some high-level information in this section for those modern men who are interested. Some of us may already be aware that when a woman's water breaks, signaling the onset of labor, her amniotic fluid is the "water" that is breaking. It is mainly made up of water from the expecting mother's body, but by the time the birth comes around, it largely consists of the baby's wee, which has been building up.

Besides keeping the baby insulated from bumps, oxygenated and well hydrated, the amniotic fluid also has a perfect cocktail of nutrients, antibodies, and nutrients to help the baby grow. It also manages to ensure a stable temperature for your little one to bathe in while developing. Put another way, this pale liquid concoction is one of your little one's best friends while they are strengthening their little body and organs in preparation for their impending grand arrival.

The amniotic fluid is held in a sac that will break either just before or in the early labor stages. When that happens, the contents will evacuate via the vagina, as many of us have seen in Hollywood films. It is worth being aware that there is a risk of infection after it breaks, and so you should help your lady seek medical attention shortly after. This will be made abundantly clear in your prenatal training.

Your Lady's Body Part 2

We have been a little preoccupied with the development and achievements of the apple of your eye during this chapter. It is worth remembering that your lady will also be undergoing a lot of her own development and changes during the second trimester. Several potential pregnancy-related symptoms or ailments are discussed in earlier chapters, but we cover some of the middle and later-stage items for consideration in the following section.

In the first trimester, we mentioned the possibility of sore nipples. However, during the second trimester, there is also a chance of having leaking nipples. This is completely normal and can start happening as early as week 14, when the woman's breasts begin producing milk. Your lady may start to notice marks on her bra, which could be early traces of colostrum. Colostrum is the secretion from a mother's breasts to feed her baby. It is packed full of nutrients and good stuff to support the baby's development. If the leaking becomes a nuisance, it is very simple to pick up some absorbent pads to deal with this.

Headaches during pregnancy are not uncommon. This can be triggered by dehydration or the impact of strong hormones that ebb and flow during the period. The best defense is to make sure your lady is drinking a minimum of eight glasses of water or fluid a day, staying well-rested and relaxed (including getting enough sleep), and maintaining a healthy diet.

However, if a headache persists for more than three hours and (pregnancy friendly) over-the-counter pain relief is ineffective, this could be a symptom of high blood pressure associated with gestational hypertension or pre-eclampsia. If your lady is exhibiting these symptoms, please help her see a healthcare professional. Typically pregnancy-related hypertension will dissipate within weeks of birth, but pre-eclampsia is more complicated.

Pre-eclampsia is a condition that typically becomes apparent after 20 weeks of pregnancy. It manifests itself via high blood pressure and damage to key organs, such as the kidneys and liver. What is unusual about it, is that it can occur in women with normal blood pressure prior to the pregnancy. Earlier in the book, we discussed the possibility of your partner experiencing swelling of the ankles and other joints that are usual for a pregnancy. However, sudden or particularly drastic swelling of the feet and hands or even the face can also point to pre-eclampsia.

Pre-eclampsia is a serious condition with potentially dire consequences if left untreated. Symptoms include severe headaches, blurred or altered vision, abdominal pain, shortness of breath, excess protein in the woman's urine, nausea and vomiting, impaired liver, and decreased platelets in the bloodstream. This condition affects approximately 5%-6% of pregnant women worldwide on average.

When treating pregnancy-related headaches, healthcare professionals will typically be ok with the woman using normal pain management solutions such as paracetamol to manage headaches during pregnancy. However, be aware that painkillers that contain codeine, caffeine, and anti-inflammatory components such as ibuprofen and or aspirin, should all be avoided. This is always good to know just in case you are tasked with a selfless trip to the pharmacy.

Given the significant changes in your partner's abdomen, she may also start to experience some pain in her pelvic region. Like many pregnancy complaints, the symptoms and strength of the sensations will vary. The main condition to be aware of is pelvic girdle pain (PGP) or symphysis pubis dysfunction (SPD). The former is the more current name as the natal medical profession realized that more joints and regions are impacted by this condition than just the symphysis pubis.

Classic symptoms are triggered by stiffness and pressure on certain joints. These symptoms may include lower back pain and will most often be felt deep in the groin region. Sometimes this condition can manifest itself in clicking or grinding sensation. The pain can range from being relatively manageable to very acute and motion inhibiting. The combined sensation from these symptoms can be quite disturbing. Still, there are ways to manage it, from simple movement instructions to physical therapy, medication, alternative acupuncture, kinesiology, reflexology, and other natural therapies.

While we have touched on some of the more serious conditions to be aware of during the second trimester for your lady, there are some minor complaints that she may be susceptible to as well. For example, leg cramps are quite common from the swelling, increased load on her legs, and pressure on the joints and tendons. Similarly, some women feel strong hot flashes from the combination of increased blood flow and hormone production. While being deeply uncomfortable, these symptoms are not usually serious, but if they become pronounced or last for long periods, please check with a healthcare professional.

Similarly, some pregnant women experience a prevalence of bleeding gums while brushing their teeth. This is also triggered by increased hormones and can lead to swollen gums. Some women are more susceptible to plaque build-ups from the hormone levels, which can lead to an increased disposition to gingivitis. Long story short, help your lady look after pearly whites during this time.

One small, slightly aesthetic concern that some expecting mothers may become aware of during the second trimester is the linea nigra. This is a vertical dark line that runs from the pubic region up towards the navel. If it becomes visible, it will be visible around the fourth or fifth month of pregnancy. The linea nigra does not pose any physical health threat and will typically vanish after birth.

Second Trimester Prenatal Tests

During the second trimester, the baby has developed far enough to be able to start testing it to eliminate any development concerns. While there are likely to be frequent smaller tests of urine, blood pressure, and occasionally blood, there will be testing focused on more specific areas or potential complications through this period.

The multiple marker test (also known as the triple screen) is a blood test typically completed anytime between week 15 and week 20. This blood test is screening for chromosomal disorders such as Down syndrome or neural tube defects such as spina bifida. It can be overlayed and assessed with the first trimester tests to provide what is referred to as an "integrated screening test."

The ultrasound screening is one of the most well-known tests as it is widely used and allows expecting parents to glimpse at their little one as it is developing within the womb. While there is an early ultrasound in the first trimester, the ultrasound during the second trimester (typically done around 20 weeks) is used to examine the baby's development, anatomy, and positioning within the womb. Unless there is something to be concerned about, there may only be the 12-week and 20-week ultrasounds, with potentially a final one just before the birth.

In some cases, your lady will have a test called amniocentesis. This procedure is where a sample of amniotic fluid and cells are taken from the uterus by a syringe for analysis. This test will often be recommended for expecting mothers over 35 years old and or if they are deemed to be at higher risk of potential complications.

The types of complications they are testing for through this procedure include genetic conditions such as Down's syndrome, Edward's syndrome or cystic fibrosis, spina bifida, fetal infection, neural defects, and fetal lung health (commonly assessing if the lungs are mature enough for birth). While I am sure this will not apply to any readers, you might be curious to know that amniocentesis can take a sample of DNA to be used in a paternity test.

Amniocentesis can provide valuable insight, but it does carry several risks to be assessed. At the less severe end of the spectrum, the woman will experience leaking amniotic fluid. More serious potential risks include needle damage from drawing the sample, infection, and in the worst case, miscarriage. That said, according to the Mayo Clinic, there is a 0.1 to 0.3 percent of miscarriage from this test. Therefore, if it is required while you and your partner will be naturally anxious, it is still deemed safe and would not be recommended unless it was important for your baby's health and wellbeing.

This marks the end of our summary of the second trimester. I look forward to discussing the final act of the gestation period in the next chapter. Well done on getting this far, and although there is a lot to remember, I hope you have found it as interesting as I did.

Chapter 8

The Third Trimester

There's a shot of adrenaline rush when you realize you've hit the third-trimester mark! You can get so caught up in all the prenatal check-ups, attending to your partner's various pains and aches, and still juggling your regular work. At the end of the day, you feel so exhausted from all the endless worrying and excitement, and then it hits you: it's the third trimester. This is where all the action is packed, the home stretch, the buzzer-beater moves, and the final rally. I have become so involved in the process of pregnancy that I didn't actually know what to expect when the reality of seeing my daughter became closer every day. I kind of felt excited about it, but I also learned so many things can go wrong. Maybe I am a worrier, but I couldn't show it because my wife needed all the strength I could muster.

There are so many things happening in the third trimester I thought it would be best to break it up by describing all the changes happening to the three of us: me, my wife, and the future baby. All of us were being changed by this pregnancy in one way or another. My wife and the baby were really transforming physically before my face, with the baby bump just growing every day. During the third trimester, I had to buy more flowing dresses and bigger sized shirts for my wife, who couldn't hide her pregnancy any longer. But I knew deep inside, I was also changing in some way I couldn't pin down.

Baby Growth Spurt

At week 29, the baby just keeps on growing bigger and bigger. The senses are becoming more developed as they become aware of lights, sounds, and touch. You can even place some sort of music on your partner's stomachs and hear the baby kicking away with each beat. I thought that classical music would make baby more intelligent, but I just couldn't bear hearing Mozart the whole day. My daughter had to experience some country music and vibrant, funky dose of Queen and Red Hot Chili Peppers I enjoyed. And by the constant kicking, my wife was getting, I think my little girl is going to be a rockstar.

The baby will now measure around 11 inches from head to rump at week 30, weighing in a 3 pounds. Hair is also becoming more prominent as the eyelashes and brows become fuller. Nails are starting to sprout. This might be the beginning of a girl's love for salons and nail treatment. I also noticed that the baby was moving a lot around this week. My wife could hear the kicks on one side and then harder on another. Are you restless kiddo? But these are good signs that the baby is quite alive and active.

The sense of hearing becomes keener at week 31. Aside from the music, the baby now seems to respond to her parent's voices. Maybe it's just my imagination, but I can feel my daughter kick when I try talking to her through her mom's big belly. I really like lying in that position, with my head on my wife's tummy, talking to my future daughter. It's those moments where you just feel so blessed to have created a life form growing inside another human. Take this week to really talk to your child and let them know that you are waiting excitedly for her.

Week 32 is the switch week for prenatal check-ups. If before, you just take the trip to the OB once a month, the last four weeks to the birthing will make you visit the doctor on a weekly basis. The more frequent check-ups are just a precaution to know that the baby and the mother are both doing well leading to the birthing. But it also signals for me that the start of the end of the race. The baby, at this point, is already starting to open its eyes and breathe. I can't imagine it with them being suspended in amniotic fluid. But I guess they are just practicing a whole lifetime of breathing and waking up.

At week 33, the baby will just keep on gaining and gaining more weight. There will be fewer grand movements now as the uterus becomes too cramped for the baby to move freely. The baby assumes a curled up position, with its knees drawn to its chest with legs crossed. It knows it is about to make the difficult descent, and it is bracing for that moment.

The fingernails reach full length at 34 weeks. The baby is now almost mature, with all major systems developed. But the lungs will still need to take some time before full maturity. Weighing in at 5 pounds, the baby is just waiting. At this point, your partner is going to feel some movements like labor pains, which are called Braxton-Hicks contractions. These are not true labor pains, so don't panic and rush off to the nearest hospital. These mini-contractions are not yet the real thing, but they sign that hormones are already surging in the woman's body to prepare her for birthing.

Week 35, the baby is still growing. There is a noticeable amount of fat depositing in the baby's tissues. These are important because they will keep her warm when exposed to the outside world. These fat pads on kids' cheeks are the types you want to just squeeze from cuteness. But they will actually help the baby to acclimatize to the lower temperature outside the uterus.

Week 36 is the penultimate point, the last week before the baby reaches full maturity. The baby can be seen blinking, and the brain has fully formed. You can also feel the baby's head sinking lower into the abdomen towards the pelvis, preparing for expulsion. You still want to keep the baby in at 36 weeks so that she could have fully mature lungs to be able to breathe outside her amniotic home.

And then, from weeks 37-40, the waiting game begins. All organ systems are fully developed and the baby has completed its full term. At any point during these weeks, your partner can go into labor. You have to be prepared when that happens. The doctor usually gives you a target day of delivery, exactly 37 weeks from the supposed last day of your partner's menses. But just like the weather, these are just estimates that may not go according to plan. I even think that my daughter took her time and really chose the moment when she wanted to go out. You can anticipate it all you want. But when the bag bursts, you just don't know what to do.

What's Happening to Her?

The third trimester will totally change your partner's body from the bikini model you met into a full mother. The surge of hormones all over her will make her go haywire, both in a physical and mental sense. The baby, of course, is just growing and growing inside her, pushing every organ away along the way. Every cell, every organ, every part of the woman's body will have to change for the event of birthing. These changes can definitely stress out your woman, and so you have to support her in all these. You can still be your dashing, flabby self, but your partner is going to morph right in front of you.

First, the growth of the baby is going to stretch the skin on the abdomen. You can see these as the familiar stretch marks on the woman's abdomen, red gashing lines that look like she was clawed. Some parts may also be rather darkly discolored, especially along the middle of her abdomen. Various spots and brown patches called chloasmas may appear on her face. Yes, we've seen those pictorials of fully pregnant women posing beautifully as though nothing happened except for the baby bump. Celebrities glorify their pregnancies by strutting off their smooth bellies to claim motherhood. But it isn't like that all the time. Pregnancy can really change your partner's skin and physical appearance and so you have to support her.

The breasts are also going to be swollen twice their size at the third trimester. You can even see yellow discharge coming out. This is called the colostrum and quite healthy for the baby. The breasts are preparing to feed the baby. Just a fun fact: stimulating the breast can actually induce birthing. The same hormone that makes the milk glands to eject milk may also stimulate the uterus to contract and start the birthing process.

Pregnancy is also the biggest weight gain a woman can have. An average of 12.5kg is actually put on throughout the pregnancy. This is to ensure that the baby and the mother has enough nutrition during the pregnancy. The weight is usually shed off months after the birthing but a little bit of that fat stays. Your partner may be concerned about her image at this point. But assure her always that you are going to stick by her through all these changes.

As the baby grows, the uterus can push all adjacent organs out of the way. The bladder, which sits behind the uterus, can become displaced, leading to frequent urination. The stomach above can be pushed higher, and this can cause her to experience acid reflux. Your partner's blood pressure can shoot up just from the compression of the heart or the extra volume from the water retained. Symptoms usually resolve upon childbirth but always go to the doctor when in doubt.

Memorable Activities

The third trimester kicks off several important preparatory events you should be mindful of. I didn't know what a baby shower was. I don't even know there was such a thing as birthing classes. I just thought that a woman should be given the privacy to give birth on her own. I was taking my woman to prenatal check-ups monthly and that should have been enough. But when friends and family started asking questions on "What should I give for the baby shower?" or "How many sessions of birthing classes have we attended?" I figured I was missing out on something. My wife was so excited about planning all these and I didn't have a clue.

So for one, my first experience of a baby shower was quite alright. I was skeptical because the idea of a party for an unborn baby wasn't something practical for me. Why not just give presents when the baby is there? But my wife was able to pull a pretty decent baby shower off. I helped of course, with all the food and logistics. Her sister took care of the program, luckily. I wasn't too sold, but my wife was just so into it, I figured it meant something special to her. It wasn't the sort of party where people got drunk silly, and I wasn't used to that. We invited over some close friends and family over lunch. Cliché as it may seem, but the theme was pink, from the decors and table mats to the balloons and invitations. Heck, there was even pink lemonade!

I was just sitting queasily in a corner, not knowing what would actually happen in a baby shower. But when people started coming in, bringing food and gifts, I began to see the point of it all. It wasn't a party for my unborn daughter, it was a party for us, especially for my wife. Being surrounded by people who were telling us, "You're going to be great parents" or "The baby should look like the both of you," really does something to me. These people are here to cheer us on our way to becoming the parents we hope to become. With all the pieces of advice on burping the baby or knowing a cry meant a change of diapers or breastfeeding time, people were telling us they were there to support us in this important chapter in our lives. I never thought much about these parties, but on that day, I just felt I wanted to be the best husband and father for my family because many people are there to support us.

The second preparation for first-time parents is supposed to be attending birthing classes. We entered this dingy room, and then there were about five couples, all heaving and moaning on the ground. I honestly thought we stumbled upon a sex cult in one of their rituals. But my wife told me we were late. We took the yoga mat at the back of the room. I was ready to bolt out, when the instructor said, "Welcome to birthing class! Please sit behind your partner."

If it wasn't for my wife's insistence, I would have definitely walked out. But as we were doing all the breathing in and out exercises for a while, I began to relax. It's not such a bad idea after all. If this meant something for my wife, then I just have to go along with it. But the more I listened to the instructor, the more I helped my wife go through the heaving and puffing of birthing, the more I realized it was actually pretty cool. You're just like rehearsing an act so that on Showtime, you'd be giving the best performance of your life. But seriously, these classes are designed to help first-time mothers and fathers to anticipate everything that may happen during childbirth. Birthing is not as natural as I assumed most women know. There was actually a proper way of pushing the baby out. For example, the woman should only push out when there is a contraction felt. If she keeps pushing and pushing for hours without contractions, she will easily tire out and wouldn't have the energy to push when the real one comes. I guess these classes allow the anxieties of childbirth to be released as you simulate the act of birthing and see how we would react to it.

Aside from supporting my wife, I actually don't know what benefit I would get from birthing classes. I mean, she would be doing all the work come that point. The classes were supposed to help her. But the instructor insisted that the classes were strictly for couples. No woman was without a partner. I was kind of bummed at that and awkward, surrounded by strange women all moaning and pushing through the exercises. What was I doing here? But as my wife got into the drama of pushing and heaving, complete with moans, I figured this was the closest thing to the birthing I would ever get. Thankfully, I would never experience the pain of giving birth. But this was my daughter too. I couldn't share in my wife's pain, but at least in these classes, I can share in her anxiety. I don't know if that counts, but I feel for my wife, and my love for her increased. Attending the class was the least that I could do.

There are many other traditions you can start with your partner on preparing for childbirth. Baby showers and birthing classes are just some of the common ones. If you want something simpler, you can perhaps try shopping with your partner for some baby clothes. Or spend an afternoon just thinking of names. I thought that birthing was a thing women were only concerned with. But there is just a part of you as a father who wants to participate somehow in that birthing process, even if it is impossible to do so in a physical way. The past 36 weeks were not just changing my wife and my daughter; it was also changing me in some way. I could never wrap the idea that I was going to be a father in my head. These traditions actually helped me embrace that role. Going through the motions of buying clothes made me even closer to my wife. I am not very comfortable with feelings and all that fuzzy stuff. But birthing was making me love my family more.

Chapter 9

The Big Day

There were many things that went wrong on the big day. This book was primarily written for all other husbands not to imitate me. Even with the best preparation, there are so many things that can go wrong. You want to be that perfect father and husband on the big day, but there are so many factors that will spoil the best laid out plans. Maybe it's just the anxiety or the excitement that clouds the decision-making, but you can't be faulted for being too concerned, can you? I hope you learn something from reading my various mishaps so when the big day comes for you, the both of you will know exactly what to do. I have arranged all these learnings in numerical format so that you could follow the drama better.

The Big Day Has No Exact Date

My wife was supposed to give birth on November 14 but the doctor told us the actual birthing could be a week earlier or later than the target date. By November 7, I was already ready to go to the hospital. For weeks, I was already planning the route we were going to take to the hospital. I even suggested that we should get checked in earlier so that we didn't have to worry about being caught unaware. But the hospital told us they could only admit patients who were already in the process of labor. I kept asking my wife if she was feeling contractions, if her bag broke, if she was feeling any pain at all. She only told me "That's cute of you, but no, it's not yet time." Days went by with November 14 being an uneventful day. Every single sound startled me, because I was always imagining that the contractions would be happening at any time. But when November 21 passed without an event, I felt bummed. The excitement turned to worry since I heard it wasn't good if my wife delivered beyond her due date. Women are actually given 40 weeks to deliver and beyond that, the baby might experience complications like eating their own faeces.

Because my daughter wasn't interested in going out soon, I took the time to launder our clothes a few streets away from our house. If this was going to last another week, we badly needed new clothes. So I was in the middle of the second cycle of washing when my phone rang.

"Honey, the bag broke."

It usually took me around 20 minutes to go from the laundry shop to the house. But when I heard that call, it only took me 5 minutes. I didn't know how many traffic rules I violated but that call just made me push that gas to full acceleration. I left the laundry at the shop and I got to the house panting. You really don't know when the big day will come, no matter how much you prepare for it.

Have a Handy Emergency Bag

My wife was leaking in the living room by the time I arrived. She was in pain, but she was trying to remain cool. I took her inside the car as soon as I carefully and as quickly as I could. I was really panicking at that time that I just eased my wife in the back seat, locked the door and took off. She was heaving at the back of the car when she shouted: "The clothes! We forgot the clothes!"

In my panic, I didn't grab the clothes we were supposed to bring for this big day. We already prepared some clothes for the hospital stay. I also forgot some documents including her prenatal check-up imaging and laboratory results. But those were the least of my concerns. I just had to get my wife to the hospital at the quickest possible time. I want my daughter to be born in the hospital and not in the car.

Looking back, we should have a handy emergency bag with all the stuff we need in one corner of the house. Maybe even better if it's in your car so that you will only have to worry about the trip to the hospital instead of the logistical concerns. But the adrenaline is amazing, looking back. I knew I was justified for speeding along byways because my wife is going to deliver. The whole 9 months was preparing me for this one crucial ride.

Be Calm

When we arrived at the hospital, they said that she was 4cms dilated and was on her way to delivering the baby. I knew that the act of delivering must have been excruciating for my wife who opted for a spontaneous vaginal delivery. I was lucky enough to be allowed in the delivery room with her. It must have been a bloody affair as a whole human being emerged from her organs. But the mental pain of waiting maybe as excruciating. In my anxiety, several thoughts were running in my head:

"What if the vaginal delivery didn't work out? What if they had to do CS?"

"Was my daughter going to be normal? What if she had missing fingers or an enlarged head? The ultrasound findings from her prenatal check-ups were unremarkable, but you never know when the baby is actually there?"

"Is my wife ok? Is she in pain?"

"Did I turn off the stove? Did I lock the doors?"

"Should I call my parents and in-laws? Shall I alert everyone?"

"What if something goes wrong?"

The takeaway here is that we just have to get through the agony of waiting for your healthy child. It's this part of birthing that is exclusively reserved for fathers. The unique experience is something we will all have to go through. However much you cope with it, whether it is drinking coffee, pacing around the hallway, calling friends, or simply sitting quietly in a corner, waiting for your baby is that one unique first time father experience we will all have. Relish it for all the nerves, the anxiety, the excitement, the bombardment of thoughts and hopes it brings. It was in waiting that I felt most weak because I cannot help my wife in any way except for being beside her. I just felt that things were not in my control anymore and I guess that is part of being a husband and a father. I will be the provider for all our lives as a family. But at this moment, I have to wait.

Document everything

For all the nine months of waiting, running thru and fro to the doctor's clinic, getting thru contraction scares and worries of childbirth mishaps, the look on my wife's face was so worth it. She's a champion, with almost 5 hours of labor and excruciating pain. I was told they were already contemplating a Caesarean section, but at the last minute, the baby just came through. My wife was exhausted, but her smile at giving birth was just priceless.

And that bundle of joy! I cannot believe I made this creature, so tiny and cute. In tears, I carried the baby for the first time. It was a hefty 7.5 lbs but I just felt the weight of a thousand hopes and dreams on my shoulder. I may have been a lousy husband and a bum man, but carrying my daughter just made me realize I wanted to change for her. I am a father, can you believe that?!

I'm glad that I document these priceless moments. I had to ask the nurse to take a picture of us together. I will always treasure that moment that my family became complete.

Conclusion

Joanne is a cute brute. Maybe it was the rock songs that I made her listen to, but she could really cry aloud. My wife and I took turns waking up at the middle of the night whenever Joanne would cry. It was either her diapers were soiled or she just needed milk. She would bawl out her eyes dry until I was able to change her diapers or her mom silenced her with milk. And then peace would return to our household. Joanne is a brute, but she is also our angel. I like looking at her sleep, her tiny chest heaving up and down. I still can't believe I deserve to be a father to this angel, but I am going to do my darn best to give her everything she wants. Sure, perhaps in the future, she's going to be a heartbreaker with her adorable lips and nose and her angelic smile. In her teenage years, she might be a stubborn student leader or an Olympic Gold Medalist. Perhaps she is going to give me a lot of problems and joys in the future. But for now, she is my daughter, my first child, the reason for my happiness. I look at my wife and I can only feel more love as she bore all those pains to make our family complete.

And so I guess, each one of us first-time-fathers are going to have our own journeys to fatherhood. We will all make mistakes, I'm sure of it. And perhaps on your second, third and the rest of your children, you will have an easier time since you know the drill. But it's the first time that is most special because you are just clueless on what to do. Don't fret or doubt yourself. Prepare as much as you can. But at the end of the day, you just have to trust that things will just fall in place. You may attend all the birthing classes, read every pregnancy preparation book and talk to every father and still feel unprepared. It's ok. We all go through that phase and I wouldn't trade that for anything. But hopefully, this book has helped prepare just a little bit better than I did. These tiny steps you take in order to make the big day as smooth and safe as possible will go a long way. Hopefully, my journey has made you still believe that being a father is worth all that trouble.

I'm so happy to have written this because there are not a lot of books out there for fathers experiencing their first babies. Sure, the more dramatic parts are reserved for the woman and they'd need all the help they can get. But I think pregnancy and childbirth are not only the responsibilities of the woman. You are just as involved as your partner in making sure that the fruit you have created becomes as healthy, as fully-developed and as well-taken cared of as possible. Pregnancy and childbirth also changes you in more ways than you can imagine. This is hard to see since the changes you will undergo are not physical and not obvious at all. The fatherly instinct, that acceptance that you are a father, can be a quiet moment for all of us. It hit me during the baby shower, while being pressured by family and friends on making sure I know how to put on a diaper. The 'I am actually a father' moment can hit you when you are just driving your wife to the clinic, seeing the sonogram of your child for the first time, buying baby clothes or even at the moment of childbirth. But it will happen to all of us. Remember that magic moment especially when you feel anxious or down about your family life. You are a father now, congratulations. But the real work of fatherhood does not end in childbirth; it only signals the start of a lifetime bearing that title. You are a father forever. We may be lousy at times when it comes to that. But let that father moment push you to become the best that you can be.

Happy Father's Day!

References

Bjorkman, D. (2020, June 10). What partners should know: The first trimester. Retrieved December 19, 2020, from https://www.mother.ly/love/what-dad-should-knowthe-first-trimester

NCT (National Childbirth Trust). (2019, October 01). What to eat when pregnant: The truth and the myths. Retrieved December 19, 2020, from https://www.nct.org.uk/pregnancy/food-and-nutrition/what-eat-when-pregnant-truth-and-myths

NCT (National Childbirth Trust). (2019, July 16). What not to eat when you're pregnant: A quick guide. Retrieved December 19, 2020, from https://www.nct.org.uk/pregnancy/food-and-nutrition/what-not-eat-when-youre-pregnant-quick-guide

5 Tips For Drinking All The Water You Need While Pregnant. (n.d.). Retrieved December 19, 2020, from https://www.mustelausa.com/drinking-water-while-pregnant

Rosenberg, J. (2020, November 09). Ten Ways to Take
Care of Yourself in Pregnancy • Midwifery Today.
Retrieved December 19, 2020, from
https://midwiferytoday.com/mt-articles/ten-ways/

Pregnancy and fish: What's safe to eat? (2019, July 13).
Retrieved December 19, 2020, from
https://www.mayoclinic.org/healthy-
lifestyle/pregnancy-week-by-week/in-
depth/pregnancy-and-fish/art-20044185

You and your pregnancy at 1 to 3 weeks. (n.d.).
Retrieved December 19, 2020, from
https://www.nhs.uk/conditions/pregnancy-and-
baby/1-2-3-weeks-pregnant/

Morning sickness: 10 tips to relieve it. (n.d.). Retrieved
December 19, 2020, from
https://www.medicalnewstoday.com/articles/37757

Listeria infection. (2020, January 18). Retrieved
December 19, 2020, from
https://www.mayoclinic.org/diseases-
conditions/listeria-infection/symptoms-causes/syc-
20355269

Weiss, R., PhD. (n.d.). Battle Anemia During Pregnancy With Iron-Rich Foods in Your Diet. Retrieved December 19, 2020, from https://www.verywellfamily.com/iron-rich-foods-to-battle-anemia-in-pregnancy-2757517

Johnson, T. C. (2020, June 12). Folic Acid Benefits in Pregnancy. Retrieved December 19, 2020, from https://www.webmd.com/baby/folic-acid-and-pregnancy

Folic Acid. (2020, November 17). Retrieved December 19, 2020, from https://www.cdc.gov/ncbddd/folicacid/index.html

General Information About NTDs, Folic Acid, and Folate. (2018, April 11). Retrieved December 19, 2020, from https://www.cdc.gov/ncbddd/folicacid/faqs/faqs-general-info.html

Pregnancy diet: Focus on these essential nutrients. (2019, December 19). Retrieved December 19, 2020, from https://www.mayoclinic.org/healthy-

lifestyle/pregnancy-week-by-week/in-
depth/pregnancy-nutrition/art-20045082

Pregnancy and exercise: Baby, let's move! (2019, June
15). Retrieved December 19, 2020, from
https://www.mayoclinic.org/healthy-
lifestyle/pregnancy-week-by-week/in-
depth/pregnancy-and-exercise/art-20046896

7 ways to look after yourself in pregnancy. (2020,
February 14). Retrieved December 19, 2020, from
https://www.tommys.org/pregnancy-information/im-
pregnant/pregnancy-news-and-blogs/7-ways-look-
after-yourself-pregnancy

Intimacy During and After Pregnancy. (2017,
November 27). Retrieved December 19, 2020, from
https://intermountainhealthcare.org/blogs/topics/live
-well/2017/11/intimacy-during-and-after-pregnancy/

Gavin, M. (Ed.). (2017, February). Taking Care of Your
Mental Health During Pregnancy (for Parents) -
Nemours KidsHealth. Retrieved December 19, 2020,
from https://kidshealth.org/en/parents/pregnant-
mental-health.html

Kaviani, M., Saniee, L., Azima, S., Sharif, F., & Sayadi, M. (2014, July). The Effect of Omega-3 Fatty Acid Supplementation on Maternal Depression during Pregnancy: A Double Blind Randomized Controlled Clinical Trial. Retrieved December 19, 2020, from https://www.ncbi.nlm.nih.gov/pmc/articles/PMC4201198/

Understand the symptoms of depression during pregnancy. (2019, October 15). Retrieved December 19, 2020, from https://www.mayoclinic.org/healthy-lifestyle/pregnancy-week-by-week/in-depth/depression-during-pregnancy/art-20237875

Hatfield, H. (n.d.). Facing Depression During Pregnancy. Retrieved December 19, 2020, from https://www.webmd.com/baby/features/facing-depression-during-pregnancy

Postpartum depression. (2018, September 01). Retrieved December 19, 2020, from https://www.mayoclinic.org/diseases-conditions/postpartum-depression/symptoms-causes/syc-20376617

Postpartum Mood Disorders. (n.d.). Retrieved December 19, 2020, from https://psychotherapy.com/mom.html

Kashtan, P. (2014, August 19). Baby Checklist: 56 Baby Essentials. Retrieved December 19, 2020, from https://www.thebump.com/a/checklist-baby-essentials

Renter, E. (2019, February 20). Preparing for a Baby? Tackle These 15 Financial Tasks. Retrieved December 19, 2020, from https://www.nerdwallet.com/blog/health/15-financial-must-dos-to-prepare-for-a-new-baby/

Fiorillo, S. (2018, December 19). How Much Does It Cost to Raise a Child in the U.S.? Retrieved December 19, 2020, from https://www.thestreet.com/personal-finance/cost-to-raise-child-14814957

Lino, M. (2020, February 18). The Cost of Raising a Child. Retrieved December 19, 2020, from https://www.usda.gov/media/blog/2017/01/13/cost-raising-child

Hoffower, H. (2019, December 09). How much it costs
to have a baby in every state, whether you have health
insurance or don't. Retrieved December 19, 2020, from
https://www.businessinsider.com/how-much-does-it-
cost-to-have-a-baby-2018-4

The Cost To Give Birth Can Vary Massively Between
Hospitals. (2014, January 25). Retrieved December 19,
2020, from https://www.huffpost.com/entry/cost-to-
give-birth_n_4617088

Rossi, H. (2014, January 16). Cost of Childbirth Varies
Widely, Without Apparent Explanation. Retrieved
December 19, 2020, from
https://www.parents.com/health/parents-news-
now/cost-of-childbirth-varies-widely-without-
apparent-explanation/

Willets, M. (2017, January 04). Interactive Map Shows
Cost of Childbirth Around the World and It's Shocking.
Retrieved December 19, 2020, from
https://www.parents.com/pregnancy/everything-
pregnancy/interactive-map-shows-cost-of-childbirth-
around-the-world-and-its/

Kashtan, P. (2014, August 19). Baby Checklist: 56 Baby
Essentials. Retrieved December 19, 2020, from
https://www.thebump.com/a/checklist-baby-
essentials

(n.d.). Retrieved December 19, 2020, from
https://www.hopkinsallchildrens.org/patients-
families/health-library/healthdocnew/a-week-by-
week-pregnancy-calendar

1st trimester pregnancy: What to expect. (2020,
February 26). Retrieved December 19, 2020, from
https://www.mayoclinic.org/healthy-
lifestyle/pregnancy-week-by-week/in-
depth/pregnancy/art-20047208

Human Chorionic Gonadotropin Hormone (HcG).
(n.d.). Retrieved December 19, 2020, from
https://www.hormone.org/your-health-and-
hormones/glands-and-hormones-a-to-
z/hormones/human-chorionic-gonadotropin-
hormone-hcg

When will I see my baby's heartbeat on an ultrasound?
(2015, July 02). Retrieved December 19, 2020, from

https://www.parents.com/pregnancy/stages/when-will-i-see-my-babys-heartbeat-on-an-ultrasound/

Marple, K. (n.d.). Growth chart: Fetal length and weight, week by week. Retrieved December 19, 2020, from https://www.babycenter.com/average-fetal-length-weight-chart

Bhargava, H. D. (2020, July 16). First Trimester of Pregnancy: What to Expect, Baby Development. Retrieved December 19, 2020, from https://www.webmd.com/baby/guide/first-trimester-of-pregnancy

Prenatal care: 1st trimester visits. (2020, August 07). Retrieved December 19, 2020, from https://www.mayoclinic.org/healthy-lifestyle/pregnancy-week-by-week/in-depth/prenatal-care/art-20044882

Second trimester: Weeks 13 to 28. (n.d.). Retrieved December 19, 2020, from https://www.tommys.org/pregnancy-information/im-pregnant/pregnancy-calendar/second-trimester-weeks-13-28

Week 13 (for Parents) - Nemours KidsHealth. (n.d.). Retrieved December 19, 2020, from https://kidshealth.org/en/parents/week13.html

Brown fat: What is it, in newborns, obesity. (n.d.). Retrieved December 19, 2020, from https://www.medicalnewstoday.com/articles/240989

Higuera, V. (2016, June 16). Vernix Caseosa: Benefits for Baby. Retrieved December 19, 2020, from https://www.healthline.com/health/pregnancy/vernix-caseosa

Preeclampsia. (2020, March 19). Retrieved December 19, 2020, from https://www.mayoclinic.org/diseases-conditions/preeclampsia/symptoms-causes/syc-20355745

Pelvic pain in pregnancy (SPD). (n.d.). Retrieved December 19, 2020, from https://www.tommys.org/pregnancy/complications/pelvic-pain-pregnancy

Linea Nigra: Pregnancy Line. (2014, August 21). Retrieved December 19, 2020, from

https://americanpregnancy.org/pregnancy-
concerns/pregnancy-line-linea-nigra/

Zoppi, L. (2018, August 23). What is Amniotic Fluid?
Retrieved December 19, 2020, from
https://www.news-medical.net/health/What-is-
Amniotic-Fluid.aspx

Fuentes, A. (Ed.). (2018, August). Prenatal Tests:
Second Trimester (for Parents) - Nemours KidsHealth.
Retrieved December 19, 2020, from
https://kidshealth.org/en/parents/tests-second-
trimester.html

Ultrasound scans. (n.d.). Retrieved December 19, 2020,
from https://www.tommys.org/pregnancy-
information/im-pregnant/antenatal-care/ultrasound-
scans

Fuentes, A. (Ed.). (2018, August). Prenatal Test:
Multiple Marker Test (for Parents) - Nemours
KidsHealth. Retrieved December 19, 2020, from
https://kidshealth.org/en/parents/prenatal-multiple-
marker.html

Amniocentesis. (2020, November 12). Retrieved December 19, 2020, from https://www.mayoclinic.org/tests-procedures/amniocentesis/about/pac-20392914

www.ingramcontent.com/pod-product-compliance
Lightning Source LLC
Chambersburg PA
CBHW051257250726
48656CB00004B/1350